Intermittent Fasting For Woman Over 50

The Ultimate Step-by-Step Guide for Senior Women to Naturally Delay Aging by Accelerating Weight Loss While Increasing Energy and Fully Detoxify the Body

[Author - Kathleen Miller]

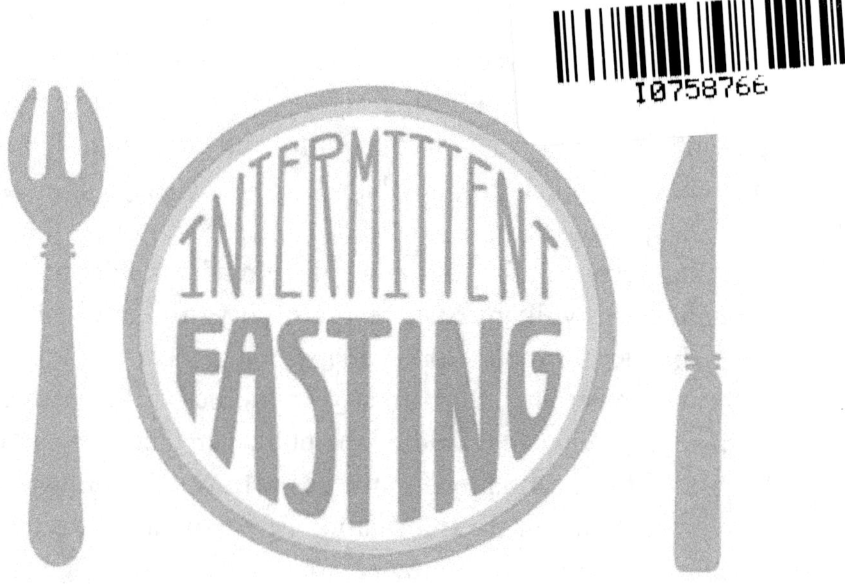

Table of Contents

INTRODUCTION

If you've read about intermittent fasting but aren't sure if it's right for you, the quick answer is: maybe. As a weight loss and fitness expert, I've been following intermittent fasting for a very time-consuming interval sieving through the science, watching displays with the hundreds of thousands of clients I've drilled, and figuring out what really works and what doesn't.

Intermittent fasting is a diet that alternates periods of eating with periods of not eating. In addition to its power to help you blast through a weight loss plateau and burn fat, there is an extraordinary list of therapeutic benefits:

Brain benefits

When my son, Grant, suffered from a severe traumatic brain injury after being in a hit-and-run accident, I explored everything that could support his recovery. Intermittent fasting combined with a ketogenic diet was an amazing grouping that made a huge difference in helping to heal his brain.

Slows aging

Intermittent fasting mimics caloric restriction, which is the most effective way we know of to surge life span. When you fast, it gives your cells the ability to detox and recycle, so your body can slow down aging and even prevent age-related diseases.

Fights cancer

Studies have shown that fasting can prevent cancer and even slow or stop its progression! It can also kill cancer cells while boosting the immune system.

If the above aren't enough to get you motivated about the possibilities of intermittent fasting, here are some more benefits: It increases insulin sensitivity, decreases the risk of cardiovascular disease, boosts energy, and enhances mental focus.

Some people believe it's not necessarily what you eat but when you eat it that matters. Those who practice intermittent fasting (IF) rave about the weight-loss benefits, improved digestion and mood, and skill to crush sugar cravings.

Intermittent fasting decreases insulin levels and increases human growth hormone, which optimizes your body's ability to burn fat.

And while there are different ways to practice IF - some do the 16:8 methods, where they fast for 16 hours and eat in an eight-hour window, while others do 5:2, where they fast for two days a week and eat normally the other five - many people are confused about what accurately they should eat during their feeding window.

It's true that intermittent fasting gives you a little more freedom to eat what you want.

Since you are typically only sitting down to one or two larger meals, you can eat more calories per meal than you would if you ate three or five meals a day.

However, there are ways to optimize your intermittent fasting for weight loss. Some people make the mistake of eating as much of whatever they want, including processed junk food, during their devouring window. If you eat in a calorie surplus, especially of empty calories and processed food, it will undo all the benefits of fasting.

"For optimal results with intermittent fasting, it's important to continue to drink plenty of water and eat nutrient-dense foods during the feeding times," said by an expert in IF field.

CHAPTER 1: WHAT IS INTERMITTENT FASTING?

Intermittent Fasting (IF) refers to dietary eating arrays that involve not eating or severely restricting calories for a prolonged period of time. There are many unique subgroups of intermittent fasting each with individual variation in the duration of the fast; some for hours, others for day(s). This has become an extremely popular topic in the science society due to all of the potential benefits on fitness and health that are being discovered.

Fasting, or periods of voluntary abstinence from food has been practiced throughout the world for ages. Intermittent fasting with the ambition of improving health relatively new. Intermittent fasting involves hindering intake of food for a set period of time and does not include any changes to the actual foods you are eating. Presently, the most common IF protocols are a daily 16 hours fast and fasting for a whole day, one or two days per week. Intermittent fasting could be considered a natural eating pattern that humans are built to implement and it traces all the way back to our Paleolithic hunter-gatherer ancestors.

The current model of a planned program of intermittent fasting could potentially help improve many aspects of health from body configuration to longevity and aging.

Although IF goes against the norms of our culture and common daily routine, the science may be pointing to less meal frequency and more time fasting as the optimal alternative to the normal breakfast, lunch, and dinner model. Here are two common myths that pertain to intermittent fasting.

Myth 1 - You Must Eat 3 Meals Per Day: This "rule" that is common in Western society was not developed based on evidence for improved health, but was adopted as the common pattern for settlers and eventually became the norm. Not only is there a lack of scientific rationale in the 3 meal-a-day model, modern studies may be showing less meals and more fasting to be optimal for human health. One study showed that one meal a day with the same amount of daily calories is better for weight loss and body composition than 3 meals per day. This finding is a basic concept that is extrapolated into intermittent fasting and those choosing to do IF may find it best to only eat 1-2 meals per day.

Myth 2 - You Need Breakfast, It's The Most Important Meal of the Day: Many false claims about the absolute need for a daily breakfast have been made. The most common claims being "breakfast increases your metabolism" and "breakfast decreases food intake later in the day". These claims have been refuted and studied over a 16-week period with results showing that skipping breakfast did not decrease metabolism and it did not increase food intake at lunch and dinner.

It is still feasible to do intermittent fasting protocols while still eating breakfast, but some people find it easier to eat a late breakfast or skip it altogether and this common myth should not get in the way.

Intermittent fasting has become quite the phenomenon these days. Recent studies showed that people who tried it have lost weight, increased health, and believed to have a long existence. Basically, intermittent fasting is a pattern of eating that alternates between periods of fasting, usually consuming only water, and non-fasting, usually eating anything a person want no matter how fattening. In other words, a person can eat anything he wants during a 24-hour period and fast for the next 24 hours.

This methodology to weight control seems to be supported by science, as well as religious and cultural practices around the globe. Adherents of intermittent fasting claim that this practice is a way to become more circumspect about food.

There are many different popular intermittent fasts and hundreds more possible variations. There are two kinds of intermittent fasts that are most basic and frequently used. First is the regular fasting in which the person only gets to eat once every 20-28 hours within a 4-hour period. The second is fasting for 1-3x a week, also called alternate day fasting, in which a person eats anything he wants on one day and fast the whole of next day.

Intermittent fasting has many beneficial effects as tested on animals like rodents and primates. One study found that there has been a "reduced serum glucose and insulin levels and increased resistance of neurons in the brain to excitotoxicity stress". In 2008, a study on intermittent fasting showed that lifespan increases of 40.4% and 56.6% in C. elegance for alternate day (24 hour) and two-of-each-three day (48 hour) fasting, respectively, as compared to an ad libitum diet. And a 2009 study showed that intermittent fasting on rats improved long-term survival after chronic heart failure via pro-angiogenic, anti-apoptotic and anti-remodeling effects.

Scientists caution that only a few studies have been done on humans who are practicing intermittent fasts. The effects of exercise and meal frequency on body composition are an interesting but largely unexplored area of research. However, there are some positive results. Just last month, the Measures of the National Academy of Sciences published a study showing that reducing calories 30% a day increased the memory function of the elderly.

In 2007, the journal Free Radical Biology & Medicine published a study that showed asthma patients who fasted had fewer symptoms, better airway function and a decrease in the markers of inflammation in the blood than those who didn't fast.

Several times have heard from people that Intermittent fasting – isn't that starvation? Lol… it's quit a funny question it's actually a good question to ask before going to (IF)

NO. Fasting differs from starvation in one crucial way: control. Starvation is the involuntary absence of food for a long time, leading to severe suffering or even death. It is neither deliberate nor controlled.

Fasting, on the other hand, is the voluntary withholding of food for spiritual, health, or other reasons. It's done by someone who is not underweight and thus has enough stored body fat to live off. Intermittent fasting done right should not cause suffering, and certainly never death.

Food is easily available, but you choose not to eat it. This can be for any period of time, from a few hours up to a few days or with medical supervision even a week or more. You may begin a fast at any time of your choosing, and you may end a fast at will, too. You can start or stop a fast for any reason or no reason at all.

Fasting has no standard duration, as it is merely the absence of eating.

Anytime that you are not eating, you are intermittently fasting. For example, you may fast between dinner and breakfast the next day, a period of approximately 12-14 hours. In that sense, intermittent fasting should be considered a part of everyday life.

Intermittent fasting is not something queer and curious, but a part of everyday, normal life. It is perhaps the oldest and most powerful dietary intervention imaginable.

Yet somehow we have missed its power and overlooked its therapeutic potential.

Learning how to fast properly gives us the option of using it or not.

At its very core, intermittent fasting simply allows the body to use its stored energy. For example, by burning off excess body fat.

It is imperative to realize that this is normal and humans have evolved to fast for shorter time periods hours or days without detrimental health consequences.

Body fat is merely food energy that has been stored away. If you don't eat, your body will simply "eat" its own fat for energy.

Life is about balance. The good and the bad, the yin and the yang. The same applies to eating and fasting. Fasting, after all, is simply the flip side of eating. If you are not eating, you are fasting.

Here's how it works:

When we eat, more food energy is ingested than can immediately be used. Some of this energy must be stored away for later use. Insulin is the key hormone involved in the storage of food energy.

Insulin rises when we eat, helping to store the excess energy in two separate ways. Carbohydrates are broken down into individual glucose (sugar) units, which can be linked into long chains to form glycogen, which is then stored in the liver or muscle.

There is, however, very limited storage space for carbohydrates; and once that is reached, the liver starts to turn the excess glucose into fat. This process is called de-novo lipogenesis (meaning literally "making new fat").

Some of this newly created fat is stored in the liver, but most of it is exported to other fat deposits in the body. While this is a more complicated process, there is almost no limit to the amount of fat that can be created.

So, two complementary food energy storage systems exist in our bodies. One is easily accessible but with limited storage space (glycogen), and the other is more difficult to access but has almost unlimited storage space (body fat).

The process goes in reverse when we do not eat (intermittent fasting). Insulin levels fall, signaling the body to start burning stored energy as no more is coming through food. Blood glucose falls, so the body must now pull glucose out of storage to burn for energy.

Glycogen is the most easily accessible energy source. It is broken down into glucose molecules to provide energy for the body's other cells. This can provide enough energy to power much of the body's needs for 24-36 hours. After that, the body will primarily be breaking down fat for energy.

So the body only really exists in two states – the fed (insulin high) state and the fasted (insulin low) state. Either we are crediting food energy (increasing stores), or we are burning stored energy (decreasing stores). It's one or the other. If eating and fasting are balanced, then there should be no net weight change.

If we start eating the minute we roll out of bed, and do not stop until we go to sleep, we spend almost all our time in the fed state. Over time, we may gain weight, because we have not allowed our body any time to burn stored food energy.

To restore balance or to lose weight, we may simply need to increase the amount of time spent burning food energy.

That's intermittent fasting.

In essence, intermittent fasting allows the body to use its stored energy. After all, that's what it is there for. The important thing to understand is that there is nothing wrong with that. That is how our bodies are designed. That's what dogs, cats, lions and bears do. That's what humans do.

If you are eating every third hour, as is often optional, then your body will constantly use the incoming food energy. It may not need to burn much body fat, if any. You may just be storing fat.

Your body may be saving it for a time when there is nothing to eat.

If this happens, you lack balance. You lack intermittent fasting.

How Our Modern Diet Is A Problem?

It's no undisclosed that obesity is on the rise in our country.

Right now, more than one-third of all adults in the U.S. are obese, totaling a whopping 78.6 million. But obesity isn't just a problem; it's downright dangerous to the population.

Obesity raises the risk of a whole slew of unwanted health conditions, like heart disease, diabetes, stroke and even some kinds of cancer. In fact, it's actually the leading cause of preventable death in our country.

Sadly, with the modern diet the way it is, it's no surprise our society has this problem. In the last few decades, the types of food we eat as well as the amounts of food have changed dramatically. Foods are more processed, they're fried into handy, to-go packages, and they're served up in super-sized portions.

Let's take a deeper look at the modern diet, and how it's led our country's health astray.

Today's diet is drastically diverse than that of Americans just 30 or 40 years ago. Then, most food was fresh, grown nearby, and cooked at home. Now, almost everything you buy has been processed even the stuff you plan to cook at home! It comes with additives, chemicals, colorings, sugars, trans fats and tons of other ingredients you wouldn't have found just a generation or two ago.

Additionally, the consumption of sugar has risen dramatically over the past couple of decades, and the average American now consumes a shocking 22 teaspoons of sugar a day, or 25 percent of their daily caloric intake. That's up 10 percent from just 10 years ago, and 20 percent since 1970.

The main cause is processed fructose which is often added to sweeten up sodas, juices, sauces, desserts and even so-called "healthy" meals and drinks. Even kids are consuming more sugar these days, setting them up for a era of poor health and nutrition.

Changing up the fats we eat has caused a problem, too. For years, many have been made to believe that animal fats, coconut oil and other healthy saturated fats could cause heart problems. People exchanged them for processed vegetable oils like canola and corn oils that can actually cause hormonal differences and metabolic changes within your body.

Over the years, repeated use of these oils has helped perpetuate the obesity problem, and more and more people have shied away from the important, healthy and naturally-occurring fats we once used.

Moreover, the increased ingesting of vegetable and processed oils have flooded our bodies with omega-6 fats throwing off the delicate balance of fatty acids. When fatty acids aren't properly balanced, it can lead to heart disease, depression Alzheimer's, arthritis, diabetes and, in some people, even certain types of cancer. Omega-3s (the fats that come from fish and fish oil) and omega-6s need to be in balance. That means 1 serving of one, for every 1 serving of the other. Today's American eats about twice as many omega-6s as omega-3s.

Accessibility foods have hurt the American health as well. As the speed of our society has quickened, more and more people are eating on the go.

They're picking up fried, fast food and eating it in the car, they're grabbing pre-packaged snacks and drinks at the gas station, and they're eating foods that aren't made fresh or naturally. It's a trend that, while easy, cheap and appropriate, has caused much more hurt than good.

Getting Back to Basics

The real key to getting the modern diet back on track is to get back to basics. Centuries and centuries ago, cavemen didn't have obesity problems. Why? Because they ate from the earth fresh vegetables and fruits, grass-fed meats and other natural, unprocessed and untouched foods.

This diet needs to serve as inspiration for today's society. Fresh produce should be a part of every meal, and instead of avoiding fats, we need to consume plenty of good, healthy fats for our bodies to thrive on.

The so-called "low fat" phase of the 80s and 90s has caused immense damage to our country's health. Fats are vital to our body's function. In fact, for optimal health, about 50 to 80 percent of your daily calories should come from good fats! That means nuts, fish, avocado, seeds, olive oil, coconut oil, eggs and beans all things found in nature.

History Of Intermittent Fasting

Compared to traditional "dieting," fasting is simple and unambiguous. It's always been done. You already unconsciously do IF whenever you skip breakfast or dinner.

Historically, during hunter gatherer days, our dynasties were in a fasting state while seeking food.

When agriculture was established, civilization came next. But when food was scarce or seasons changed, fasting was still a way of life. Cities and castles stored grain and cured meat for the winter. Before irrigation, lack of rain meant famine, and people fasted to make their stored food last as long as possible until the rains came back and it was possible for crops to survive again.

Religions flourished in this arrangement of people living closer together, distributing and spreading belief and traditions. And religions also prescribed fasting.

Hinduism calls fasting "Vaasa" and observes it during special days or festivals, as a private penance, or to honor their personal gods. Islam and Judaism have Ramadan and Yom Kippur, when it's forbidden to work, eat, drink, wash, wear leather and have intercourse. In Catholicism, it's six weeks of fasting before Easter or before Holy Week.

CHAPTER 2: HOW INTERMITTENT FASTING WORKS

Weight loss

For the most part, people who follow the 5:2 diet plan are looking to lose weight.

To lose weight, a person typically needs to eat fewer calories than they burn. Nutritionists call this a caloric deficit.

When someone follows this correctly, the 5:2 diet may be a simple, straightforward way to cut calories, which may help burn extra fat.

While there are not many studies on the 5:2 diet specially, initial studies on intermittent fasting seem promising.

A review in the Annual Review of Nourishment noted that in animal studies, a related intermittent fasting diet led to a cutback in fat tissue and the cells that store fat.

A 2018 review and meta-analysis compared intermittent fasting to simple calorie curb diets. This research noted that intermittent fasting is as effective as calorie restriction when it comes to weight loss and successful metabolic health.

Reducing the risk of type 2 diabetes

Original studies also suggest an intermittent calorie diet may also help shrink the risk of diabetes in some people.

Research from 2014 suggests that both intermittent fasting diets and calorie restriction diets helped reduce fasting insulin levels and insulin resistance in adults who were overweight or obese. The reviewers did call for more research to confirm these findings.

This does not suggest that intermittent fasting is a better diet, just an equally effective alternative for people who find calorie restriction diets difficult.

Diet for Weight Loss

If you need to lose weight, the diet can be very effective when done right.

This is mainly because the eating pattern helps you consume fewer calories.

Therefore, it is very important not to compensate for the fasting days by eating much more on the non-fasting days.

Intermittent fasting does not cause more weight loss than regular calorie restriction if total calories are matched.

That said, fasting protocols similar to the 5:2 diet have shown a lot of promise in weight loss studies:

• A recent review found that modified alternate-day fasting led to weight loss of 3–8% over the course of 3–24 weeks.

• In the same study, participants lost 4–7% of their waist circumference, meaning that they lost a lot of harmful belly fat.

• Intermittent fasting causes a much smaller reduction in muscle mass when compared to weight loss with conventional calorie restriction.

Intermittent fasting is even more effective when combined with exercise, such as endurance or strength training.

What to Do If You Feel Unwell or Uncontrollably Hungry

During the first few fast days, you can expect to have episodes of tremendous hunger. It is also normal to feel a little weaker or slower than usual.

However, you'll be surprised at how quickly the hunger fades, especially if you try to keep busy with work or other errands.

Additionally, most people find that the fast days become easier after the first few fasts.

If you are not used to fasting, it may be a good idea to keep a small snack handy during your first few fasts, just in case you feel faint or ill. But if you repeatedly find yourself feeling ill or faint during fast days, have something to eat and talk with your doctor about whether you should continue.

Intermittent fasting is not for everyone, and some people are unable to tolerate it.

Is it safe for everyone?

The diet may be a helpful substitute to some people looking for a less restrictive diet plan, but it is not for everyone.

People who are prone to low blood sugar or easily feel dizzy or fatigued if they do not eat may not want to follow a diet that involves fasting.

Pregnant or breastfeeding women must also avoid fasting. Children and teenagers should avoid fasting unless under the direct guidance of a doctor, as their bodies are still emerging.

Anyone with a chronic condition, such as diabetes, can consult a doctor before trying any diet that includes fasting.

Who Should Avoid the Diet, or Intermittent Fasting Overall?

Although intermittent fasting is very safe for healthy, well-nourished people, it does not suit everyone.

Some people should avoid dietary restrictions and fasting completely. These include:

• Individuals with a history of eating disorders.

• Individuals who often experience drops in blood sugar levels.

• Pregnant women, nursing mothers, teenagers, children and individuals with type 1 diabetes.

• People who are malnourished, underweight or have known nutrient deficiencies.

• Women who are trying to conceive or have fertility issues.

Furthermore, intermittent fasting may not be as beneficial for some women as it is for men.

Some women have reported that their menstrual period stopped while they were following this type of eating pattern. However, things went back to normal when they returned to a regular diet.

Therefore, women should be careful when starting any form of intermittent fasting, and stop doing it instantly if any adverse effects occur.

The diet is an easy, effective way to lose weight and improve metabolic health.

Many people find it much easier to stick to than a conventional calorie-restricted diet.

If you're looking to lose weight or improve your health, the diet is definitely something to consider.

CHAPTER 3: THE SCIENCE BEHIND IT

The modern era of agriculture and factory-laden "food" (or food-like substances) has absolutely changed the way humans view and consume food on a daily basis, leading to the laundry list of health problems that our society faces today.

Although IF is an primeval practice, the science after its many health benefits is just recently being exposed to mainstream society.

When you fast, you basically allow your body to naturally cleanse, repair and regenerate itself for optimal function.

Three of the main health-promoting mechanisms associated with fasting include the metabolic regulation of circadian biology, the gut microbiome and different lifestyle behaviors.

Circadian Biology

Humans (and other organisms) have evolved to develop a circadian clock that ensures physiological processes within your body are performed at optimal times throughout the day.

These circadian rhythms occur across 24-hour light-dark cycles and influence changes in biology and behavior.

Interrupting this circadian rhythm negatively impacts metabolism which contributes to obesity and associated diseases such as type 2 diabetes, cardiovascular disease and cancer.

This is where intermittent fasting comes in.

Feeding signals seem to be the main timing cue for how your circadian rhythms function and thus control certain metabolic, physiological and behavioral pathways that contribute to overall health and longevity.

Certain behavioral interventions such as (you guessed it!) intermittent fasting can help synchronize your circadian rhythms leading to improved fluctuations in gene illustration, reprogramming of energy metabolism and improved hormonal and body weight regulation, all factors that play a vital role in optimizing your health outcomes.

The Gut Microbiome

The gastrointestinal (GI) tract, better known as the "gut," plays an extremely important role in regulating several processes within your body.

Many functions of the gut (and nearly every physiological and biochemical function in your body) are influenced by your circadian rhythm described above.

For example, gastric emptying, blood flow and metabolic responses to glucose are greater during the daytime than at night.

So, it's likely that a chronically disturbed circadian rhythm can affect gut function contributing to impaired metabolism and increased risk for chronic disease.

The gut microbiome, also known as our "second brain," has been the subject of extensive research in both health and disease due to its profound involvement in human metabolism, physiology, nutrition and immune function.

Intermittent fasting has a direct and positive influence on the gut microbiome through:

- Reduced gut permeability

- Diminished systemic inflammation

- Promotion of energy balance by enhancing gut integrity.

Research on both the gut and intermittent fasting continues to emerge while the potential for prevention and treatment of diseases is becoming more widely understood.

Lifestyle Behaviors

Intermittent fasting is shown to help modify different health performances such as caloric intake (i.e. how much you eat), energy expenditure (how much you move) and sleep.

There's no surprise that these three factors contribute to one of the biggest draws to intermittent fasting today: weight loss.

A recent study showed that increasing the nightly fasting duration to greater than 14 hours led to a significant decrease in caloric intake and weight with improvements to:

- Energy levels

- Sleep satisfaction

- Satiety at bedtime

Intermittent fasting also reduces nighttime eating, which contributes to poor sleep quality and reduced sleep duration leading to insulin resistance and increased risk of obesity, diabetes, cardiovascular disease and cancer.

Fasting puts an adaptive cellular stress on the body which in turn allows your body to cope with more severe stressors that may occur and thus protect against potential disease progressions.

This concept is known as hormesis when an exposure to a mild stress causes cells in your body to become more resilient against other, more severe stressors.

Think of it this way – what doesn't kill you really does make you stronger!

CHAPTER 4: INTERMITTENT FASTING STAGES

Whole Day Fasting

When it comes to eating programs, humans are built for suppleness. It's a complete myth that people "need" to eat three times a day (or 6 meals a day, or on any other specific schedule). Think about that for a minute: there's no way we would have survived the caveman days if we needed to eat every few hours. If we were really that fragile, we would have died off ages ago.

3 meals a day is the typical cultural pattern, but who says your particular body might not do better on some other eating schedule? Some people prefer to eat every day, but within a restricted window. Other people eat normally most of the time, but occasionally embark on long fasts.

But there's also an option in between: eat normally on some days, but then periodically go on a 24-hour fast. A common option is alternate-day fasting, but some people also do 1-3 fast days per week on set days.

The Case for One-Day Fasts

For weight loss, the idea of occasional 24-hour fasts is basically low-effort calorie reduction. Sure, most people will be hungrier and eat more on the day after their fast, but they probably won't eat twice as much as they otherwise would.

And that calorie reduction comes without the need to count the calories in anything you eat the only question is yes or no on food for the day.

This is more or less the same idea as a limited eating window (say, eating only between noon and 8pm). But some people find that cramming all their food into a short eating window gives them an upset stomach for those people, one-day fasting might be easier because on "feeding" days, you can spread out your meals normally.

In terms of benefits that aren't related to weight loss, fasting has been claimed to help with everything from cancer prevention to life extension, but most of those claims are based on animal studies, and it's not clear whether the benefits in humans live up to the hype.

In this post, we'll take a look at studies on one-day fasts and alternate-day fasting, focusing on some specific questions:

• Do regular fast days' work for weight loss?

• Do regular fast days have benefits other than weight loss?

• Are the effects different in lean vs. obese subjects?

At the end, we'll also take a look at variations on the one-day fast theme, including modified fasting.

One-Day Fasts: The Big Picture

A lot of the research on this has focused precisely on alternate-day fasting (eat on Day 1, fast on Day 2, eat on Day 3, fast on Day 4, etc.). In terms of weight loss, here's a big-picture overview of review studies:

• Alternate-day fasting is just as effective as very-low calorie diets for weight loss, but it may be easier: some patients found it simpler to fast every day than to restrict calories every day.

• Unfortunately, an alternate-day fasting scheme doesn't prevent your metabolism from fighting back against weight loss. This review looked exclusively at metabolic adaptations to weight loss. You might expect that alternate-day fasting would be superior to constant dieting here, but the study didn't actually find evidence of that – both were about the same.

As for non-weight-related benefits, the evidence in humans is mixed but encouraging:

• A 2007 review of alternate-day fasting found that it may help to improve blood lipids (higher HDL cholesterol, lower triglycerides), but also found that alternate-day fasting and ordinary calorie limitation were equally good for insulin levels and blood sugar control.

• Another study found that severe calorie restriction (less than 20% of energy needs) on alternate days reduced inflammation and oxidative stress in overweight adults with asthma.

• Finally, this study found that intermittent energy restriction (less than 25% of energy needs) reduced inflammation and improved blood lipids in overweight women.

Is it a magical cancer stoppage/cure tactic? No, but nothing really is. In overweight subjects, one-day fasts seem to reduce some measures of overall physical stress and chronic poor health.

Obese vs. Non-Obese Subjects

Some more dramatic weight-loss approaches (e.g. protein-sparing modified fasts) are fine for people with a lot of weight to lose, but don't work so well for the last 5-10 pounds. So what about occasional one-day fasts?

This analysis looked at alternate-day fasting in 16 non-obese subjects (8 men, 8 women). The subjects fasted every other day for 22 days. On average, they lost about 2.5% of their initial body weight (so a 150-pound person would lose just under 4 pounds). But they never stopped being hungry on fasting days.

Reflecting that most people don't want to be hungry every other day for the rest of their lives, this suggests that alternate-day fasting might not be the best strategy for people who are already fairly close to their target weight.

On the other hand, not everyone responds the same way. Some fairly lean people might be perfectly happy taking regular fast days. The study did show that it worked fine, just that it wasn't pleasant. If you don't notice the same amount of hunger, it might be just the thing for you.

Variations on a Theme

Most of the studies so far have been in alternate-day fasting. But the same ideas (a hormonal break from digestion, low-effort calorie reduction) still apply to vaguely less rigorous fasting proprieties like…

Fasting 1-3 days per week

The benefit: makes your social calendar easier.

One big barrier to alternate-day fasting is that most of us have a weekly schedule, and weeks have an odd number of days. Fasting every other day means that you're frequently changing the day of the week when your fast happens, which can be inconvenient. It may be easier for some people to fast on specific calendar days, rather than every other day.

Is it Worth a Try?

Probably yes if…

• You're primarily interested in weight loss, especially if you have quite a bit of weight to lose

• You don't mind the idea of going a whole day with no or very little food

• You have a lot of weight to lose.

Probably no if…

• You'd rather just eat less every day (there's no evidence that alternate-day fasting works better, so you may as well do what you prefer).

• You do very intense exercise most days or every day.

• You get unpleasant side effects (weakness, dizziness, feeling cold, etc.) from fasting. If you still want to fast in this case, you might consider the classic "intermittent fasting" design with a compressed eating window, which can be a little less intense but still has similar benefits.

Have you ever tried daily fasts? How many times a week? Did you fully fast, or did you do a modified fast?

CHAPTER 5: MYTHS ABOUT INTERMITTENT FASTING

Fasting And Autophagy

But what is autophagy? The word derives from the Greek auto (self) and phage in (to eat). So the word literally means to eat oneself. Essentially, this is the body's mechanism of getting rid of all the broken down, old cell machinery (organelles, proteins and cell membranes) when there's no longer enough energy to sustain it. It is a regulated, orderly process to degrade and recycle cellular components.

There is a related, better known process called apoptosis also known as programmed cell death. Cells, after a certain number of division, are programmed to die. While this may sound kind of macabre at first, realize that this process is crucial in maintaining good health. For example, suppose you own a car. You love this car. You have great memories in it. You love to ride it.

But after a few years, it starts to look kind of beat up. After a few more, it's not looking so great. The car is costing you thousands of dollars every year to maintain. It's breaking down all the time. Is it better to keep it around when it's nothing but a hunk of junk? Apparently not. So you get rid of it and buy a snazzy new car.

The same thing happens in the body. Cells become old and junky. It is better that they be programmed to die when their useful life is done. It sounds really cruel, but that's life. That's the process of apoptosis, where cells are pre-destined to die after a certain amount of time. It's like leasing a car. After a certain amount of time, you get rid of the car, whether it's still working or not. Then you get a new car. You don't have to worry about it breaking down at the worst possible time.

Autophagy – replacing old parts of the cell

The same process also happens at a sub-cellular level. You don't necessarily need to replace the entire car. Sometimes, you just need to replace the battery, throw out the old one and get a new one. This also happens in the cells. Instead of killing off the entire cell (apoptosis), you only want to replace some cell parts. That is the process of autophagy, where sub-cellular organelles are destroyed and new ones are rebuilt to replace it.

Old cell membranes, organelles and other cellular debris can be removed. This is done by sending it to the lysosome which is a specialized organelle containing enzymes to degrade proteins.

What activates autophagy?

Nutrient deprivation is the key activator of autophagy. Remember that glucagon is kind of the opposite hormone to insulin. It's like the game we played as kids 'opposite day'. If insulin goes up, glucagon goes down.

If insulin goes down, glucagon goes up. As we eat, insulin goes up and glucagon goes down. When we don't eat (fast) insulin goes down and glucagon goes up. This increase in glucagon stimulates the process of autophagy. In fact, fasting (raises glucagon) provides the greatest known boost to autophagy.

This is in essence a form of cellular cleansing. The body identifies old and substandard cellular equipment and marks it for destruction. It is the accumulation of all this junk that may be responsible for many of the effects of aging.

Fasting is actually far more beneficial than just stimulating autophagy. It does two good things. By stimulating autophagy, we are clearing out all our old, junky proteins and cellular parts. At the same time, fasting also stimulates growth hormone, which tells our body to start producing some new snazzy parts for the body. We are really giving our bodies the complete renovation.

You need to get rid of the old stuff before you can put in new stuff. Think about renovating your kitchen. If you have old, crappy 1970s style lime green cabinets sitting around, you need to junk them before putting in some new ones. So the process of destruction (removal) is just as important as the process of creation. If you simply tried to put in new cabinets without taking out the old ones, it would be pretty ugly. So fasting may in some ways reverse the aging process, by getting rid of old cellular junk and replacing it with new parts.

A highly controlled process

Autophagy is a highly regulated process. If it runs amok, out of control, this would be detrimental, so it must be carefully controlled. In mammalian cells, total depletion of amino acids is a strong signal for autophagy, but the role of individual amino acids is more variable. However, the plasma amino acid levels vary only a little. Amino acid signals and growth factor / insulin signals are thought to converge on the mTOR pathway sometimes called the master regulator of nutrient signaling.

So, during autophagy, old junky cell components are broken down into the component amino acids (the building block of proteins). What happens to these amino acids? In the early stages of starvation, amino acid levels start to increase. It is thought that these amino acids derived from autophagy are delivered to the liver for gluconeogenesis.

They can also be broken down into glucose through the tricarboxylic acid (TCA) cycle. The third potential fate of amino acids is to be incorporated into new proteins.

The consequences of accumulating old junky proteins all over the place can be seen in two main conditions Alzheimer's Disease (AD) and cancer.

Alzheimer's Disease involves the accumulation of abnormal protein either amyloid beta or Tau protein which gums up the brain system. It would make sense that a process like autophagy that has the ability to clear out old protein could prevent the development of AD.

What turns off autophagy? Eating. Glucose, insulin (or decreased glucagon) and proteins all turn off this self-cleaning process. And it doesn't take much. Even a small amount of amino acid (leucine) could stop autophagy cold. So this process of autophagy is unique to fasting something not found in simple caloric restriction or dieting.

There is a balance here, of course. You get sick from too much autophagy as well as too little. Which gets us back to the natural cycle of life feast and fast. Not constant dieting. This allows for cell growth during eating, and cellular cleansing during fasting balance. Life is all about balance.

CHAPTER 6: BENEFITS AND DOWNSSIDES

The benefits of intermittent fasting are vast. Fasting gets a bad rap, but there is real science behind the technique of fasting, in particular, intermittent fasting. Many people think that someone who is fasting has an eating disorder, but nothing could be farther from the truth.

The truth is that in today's society, we eat far too much and too often. Our bodies are very precise mechanisms that, allowed to run properly, will take care of us far beyond our imagination. The problem lies with the fact that historically, for thousands and thousands of years, we were a species with little food resources and we worked long and hard each and every day for the morsels we did get. Today, we have a plethora of food, most of it very fattening, and sedentary lifestyles. This both contributes to obesity and disease.

Fasting intermittently can eliminate many problems caused from overeating and sitting around all day instead of out hunting and gathering. The fact is that we have not evolved enough to be able to handle all the calories that we ingest on a daily basis, our bodies still operate as if we were hunter and gatherers. Not until the 20th century did most people have food at the ready, so 100 years is not even close to adequate time to adjust how our body operates.

Extreme blood pressure, excessive cholesterol, and obesity are all problems that can be helped with intermittent fasting. A particularly effective fasting plan is called the Fast 5. This plan requires you to fast for 19 hours every day and eat for 5 consecutive hours. It is important to note that you DO eat when fasting intermittently. Eating is essential to your health, but eating once or twice a day during a short period is more natural to our bodies than stuffing them 12 out of 24 hours in a day. Again, up until the 20th century, most people only managed to eat once a day for thousands of years.

The pattern of eating called "Intermittent Fasting" usually means one fasts for a period of time and eats for a period of time. Many choose a 24 hour cycle of fasting, then eat healthy the next day, and continue this process as a lifestyle change.

Research has been done on animals to find the benefits of this type of fasting, and you will be happy to know it really can be beneficial to your health!

Intermittent fasting can add 40%-56% more years to your life! That in itself is reason enough to do it. However other benefits include body weight reduction and fat oxidation.

When you fast your body is forced to scavenge for fuel thus removing aged and damaged cells in the process. This sort of cleanses the body of unwanted and unwanted things and helps the weight loss and benefits of the good food choices be increased and more beneficial to your body.

Rats have been shown to have long-term and improved survival after heart failure after being on an IF eating plan, too. Researchers are also saying that it might help age related deficits in cognitive function, too, so that tells me that it might help ward off Alzheimer's Disease and other types of Dementia!

Your risk of heart disease and other heart ailments may also be decreased when you start a healthy intermittent fasting regimen. Your risk for other chronic illnesses and diseases will also most likely be reduced.

A improved you can begin with intermittent fasting and healthy food choices! Keep carbs to 50-100 grams per day. Many women eat between 1200-1500 calories per day, and when limiting their carbs, they are still losing weight. Men can handle up to 2000 calories per day. Of course less is best, and you need to determine caloric intake based on your activity such as working hard and exercising.

Drink lots of fluids, especially water and exercise in the evenings if possible. This will help with those late night cravings.

Once you start eating and drinking healthier, your body won't crave as much (if any) junk food, so making healthy food choices will simply get easier and easier as you progress in the intermittent fasting routine.

Alternate Day Fasting or ADF means alternating days of eating and not eating any food, but there is also an intermittent fasting called Modified Fasting where you consume about 20% of your normal calories one day and then eat normally (but healthy) the next day. This is frequently more attainable for people because they feel less deprived when they are able to at least eat something daily, and it still has most of the benefits of the ADF regimen.

Whatever you choose to do, make sure you tell your health care professional of your plans so he or she is aware and can work with you to reach your goals. If you want to lose weight, lose fat and feel better, then intermittent fasting might be the answer for you!

The fasting periods were often called 'cleanses', 'detoxifications', or 'purifications', but the idea is similar – e.g. to abstain from eating food for a certain period of time, often for health reasons. People imagined that this period of abstinence from food would clear their bodies' systems of toxins and rejuvenate them. They may have been more correct than they knew.

Some of the purported health benefits of intermittent fasting include:

• Weight and body fat loss

• Increased fat burning

• Lowered blood insulin and sugar levels

• Possibly reversal of type 2 diabetes

• Possibly improved mental clarity and concentration

• Possibly increased energy

• Possibly increased growth hormone, at least in the short term

• Possibly an improved blood cholesterol profile

• Possibly a reduction in the risk of Alzheimer's disease

• Possibly longer life

• Possibly activation of cellular cleansing by stimulating autophagy

• Possibly reduction of inflammation.

Fasting offers many important unique advantages that are not available in typical diets.

Where diets can complicate life, intermittent fasting may simplify it. Where diets can be expensive, intermittent fasting can be free. Where diets can take time, fasting saves time. Where diets may be limited in their availability, fasting is available anywhere. And as discussed earlier, fasting is a potentially powerful method for lowering insulin and decreasing body weight.

Common Downside Mistakes When It Comes to Intermittent Fasting

The concept of intermittent fasting seems fairly honest. You withhold from eating in intervals somewhere between 16 or 20 hours a day or heavily restrict your intake and eat a very low-calorie diet a couple day a week. There are also some IF followers who eat just one meal a day (also called OMAD).

There's quite a bit of research proving that IF works for weight loss and improves things like blood sugar control and cholesterol, which are indicators for chronic diseases. Some studies have even found that IF may boost people's energy and help them sleep better.

I've been a dietitian for so many years, so I've read my share of research on IF, I've written about it a handful of times, and I've even tried intermittent fasting out for myself. Here's my take: it works really well for some people regardless of what "type" of IF they follow, but one common denominator is that plenty of folks out there are doing it wrong.

There happens to be a lot of misinformation floating around the internet (both about intermittent fasting and dieting as a whole category), so I culled a list of some of the top comments and questions on Reddit's Intermittent Fasting drift and answered them the best I could. Here are some common questions I found about IF, plus some common faults to avoid when trying it.

Some people come into difficulty with Intermittent Fasting because they approach it in the wrong way, being aware of the right procedures when undertaking Intermittent Fasting can be the difference between success and failure.

Here are the top mistakes that I see people making all the time when they are fasting:

1. You're jumping into intermittent fasting too fast.

The biggest reason most diets fail is because they're such an extreme departure from our common, natural way of eating that they often feel impossible to maintain. Just a thought, but if you're new to IF and are familiar to eating every two hours on the hour, maybe don't throw yourself into a hard-core 24-hour-fast from hell.

If you're adamant about the concept of fasting, start with some beginners 12/12 method where you're fasting for 12 hours per day and eating within the 12-hour window. That's probably pretty close to what you're used to doing anyway, and who knows, it might be the only (if even that) defensible way to follow along.

2. You're choosing the wrong plan for your lifestyle.

Again, don't set yourself up for misery by signing up for something you know is going to cramp your style. If you're a night owl, don't plan to start your fast at 6 p.m.

If you're a daily gym-goer who Instagram's their WOD every morning and aren't willing to sacrifice your daily Spin, don't choose a plan that severely restricts calories a few days a week.

3. You're eating too much during the eating window.

This one is the most common trap I would expect to see people fall into with IF. If you've chosen a particularly obstructive regimen that's left you hangry AF for hours of the day, the moment the clock says "it's time to eat," you're likely to go a wee bit overboard. Research suggests restrictive diets often don't work because we tend to become so emotionally (and physically) starved that when we do allow ourselves to eat, we go hog wild and overeat in a fit of deprivation. Any diet that has you preoccupied with your next meal is a recipe for a binge so make sure you're not allowing yourself to feel unnecessarily hungry for long periods of time.

4. You're not eating enough during the eating window.

Yep, not eating enough is also legit cause of weight gain, and I'll tell you why. In addition to setting yourself up for a rebound similar to what we deliberated with the last common IF mistake, not eating enough cannibalizes your muscle mass, causing your metabolism to slow.

Without that metabolic muscle mass, you may be sabotaging your ability to maintain (never mind to lose) fat in the future. The challenge with IF is that because you're eating according to some arbitrary temporal rules, rather than listening to your body's innate cues, it's really difficult to know your true needs.

If you're adamant about doing the diet, be sure to speak to a registered dietitian to help you assess and meet your nutrient needs safely.

5. Using it as an excuse to eat rubbish.

Unfortunately, people think that intermittent fasting is a magic pill that will solve all their problems. Yes, it is an incredibly effective tool to take control of your health but it won't cancel out eating a diet full of processed foods and sugar. When you are intermittent fasting it is even more important to nourish your body with nutrient dense, whole foods.

When you are in the fasted state, your body starts to break down damaged components and then uses them for of energy, this process cleans and heals the body. It also means your body becomes more sensitive to the food you eat, this is great if it's full of nutrients to nourish the body, but not good if you are eating rubbish.

Not only that, if you aren't nourishing yourself with nutrient dense foods, you will feel hungry all the time – your body will crave nutrients.

6. You're Eating Too Many Calories.

"Does anyone else eat like crazy right when the fast is over and is it normal to have a huge appetite during the feeding period? It is hard for me to get full after a 20 hour fast and I just eat the whole 4 hours. LOL."

I'd venture to guess that this person is eating more calories than what's needed in that 4-hour window. So instead of laughing your way through a marathon all-you-can-eat session, plan for how you'll break your fast. Stock up on high-protein foods (like meats and seafood) and/or high-fiber foods (like fruits, vegetables, beans, and most whole grains). They'll not only fill you up, but will keep you feeling full.

"If I do a 20:4 fast then I should consume 1500-2000 calories within four hours? Am I understanding this correctly?"

Technically, yes. But depending on a person's body size, eating 2,000 calories in a 4-hour window might not yield any weight loss. I don't know this person's size, though. Now, most people lose weight on 1,500 calories, but one of the pros of IF is that it's hard to eat a ton of calories in a short window of time.

For some, following IF is an easier way to cut calories and lose weight than simply following a traditional calorie-restricted diet. So if you can't hit the 1,500- or 2,000-calorie mark in 4 hours every day, it's OK. If falling below 1,200 calories a day becomes a regular habit, though, reconsider your diet plan. If you're not sure how many calories you're consuming, track them in a free app like MyFitnessPal.

7. You're Overanalyzing.

"Does IF mean no food outside meal times, or no calories?"

Um, they are one in the same, no? Does anyone reading this article know of foods that have zero calories? If so, please share! This person's assumption is correct, though—no food and no calories outside of the "feeding window."

Does anyone else feel like this question comes up about a thousand times a day? Short answer: Yes. Eating anything with calories breaks your fast.

Exceptions to this rule would be black coffee, unsweetened and milk-free tea, water, and diet soda (though research says diet soda could actually increase your appetite, which might make it hard to stick to your fast.)

8. You're Pushing Yourself Too Hard.

"I've been doing IF almost 2 months, mostly OMAD, sometimes 48/72 hours extended fasts. The last 3 or 4 days whenever I break my fast I feel a great regret. I always feel like I could push the fast a little longer. What should I do?"

Extending a fast doesn't supercharge the powers of IF. If this sounds familiar to you, please find yourself a counselor who specializes in eating disorders.

I'm not saying you, or this person here, has an eating disorder, but food should not induce feelings of remorse or regret. Left untreated, this could develop into a larger problem. And also, huge kudos to this person for so bravely speaking up and sharing their food feelings!

9. Attempting to do too many things at once – over train, under eat and try fasting.

If you have spent a number of years eating badly and not exercising and you would like to try IF, don't bite off more than you can chew (pun intended!) at the start. Ease yourself into fasting and training gradually; don't start training five times per week, fasting every day and restricting calories when you do eat from day one.

The combination can lead to problems. Your body thrives with a little bit of physical stress here and there but too much stress can create chronic issues.

10. You're not drinking enough.

Your intermittent fasting regimen might have you refraining from food, but water should always be nearby, especially since you're missing out on the hydration you often get from foods like fruits and veggies. Dehydration can lead to muscle cramps, headaches, and exacerbate hunger pangs, so always make sure you're sipping H2O between (and during) feasts.

Followed all the rules and still struggling? It's not you; it's likely the diet. Research suggests that intermittent fasting has a 31 percent dropout rate, while research on diets in general suggests that as much as 95 percent of diets fail.

Try to focus more on what your body tells you, rather than what the clock says, and you're much more likely to get the nutrition your body needs.

11. Giving Up Too Soon.

Intermittent fasting takes a certain amount of discipline, but as mentioned above, it also takes time to get used to. The first four to five days are definitely the hardest. You will feel hungry.

You might feel lightheaded or exhausted or get headaches. Know that those feelings quickly pass and by the end of the first week, your body will start to adapt.

Your hunger will actually diminish and you'll start to feel more energetic and more focused. If you don't feel better after the first week, you may be doing too much too soon, or you may have chosen a plan that doesn't work for you.

CHAPTER 7: 5 WAYS TO DO INTERMITTENT FASTING

It isn't complicated, either. There are just 5 simple steps to getting started:

Let's take a look at each.

Step 1. Choose which protocol you want to follow.

Intermittent fasting has really taken off in recent years, and there are several popular schedules to choose from.

The ones you'll hear the most about in fitness circles are Leangains, Eat Stop Eat, The Warrior Diet, and alternate-day fasting.

There are many others, of course, but all that I've seen are just derivatives of the above, and thus aren't worth mentioning.

Let's take a closer look at each of those above, and see what will best fit your needs.

Leangains is an intermittent fasting diet created and popularized by Martin Berkhan.

It was designed specifically for weightlifters and people who care about their body composition, and it's why IF has gained so much traction in the bodybuilding section.

It's also my personal favorite out of the bunch because it's simple, effective, and doesn't involve tremendously long fasts.

Here's how it works:

• Men should fast for 16 hours and eat all food in the other 8 hours of the day. Women should fast for 14 hours and eat food in the remaining 10 hours.

• The fast starts after you've eaten your last meal of the day, and ends with your first meal of the day.

• You aren't supposed to eat or drink any calories during the fast, but black coffee, zero-calorie sweeteners, diet soda, and sugar-free gum are allowed.

So, for example, if you're a man and you eat your last meal at 9 PM at night, then you won't eat your next meal until 1 PM the following day. If you're a woman, you break your fast two hours' sooner, at 11 AM.

As you can see, Leangains more or less boils down to "skip breakfast," which many people like to do anyway.

Step 2. Calculate your calories.

You may have heard that you don't have to watch your calories with intermittent fasting.

This is absolutely false.

No matter what type of diet you follow, caloric intake is always king.

If you want to lose weight, you need to eat fewer calories than you burn, and if you want to gain weight, you need to eat more.

End of story.

That said, intermittent fasting may help you better control your caloric intake by making the overall experience of dieting more enjoyable. The better you can stick to the plan, the better your results will be in the long run.

Step 3. Calculate your macronutrients.

You've probably heard that not all calories are identical. That "a calorie isn't a calorie."

This isn't true if all you want to do is loss or gain weight.

If, however, you want to lose fat and not muscle (or gain muscle and not fat), then it's very true. Some calories are more important than others.

For example, …

• Eating enough protein helps you better recover from your workouts, preserve muscle while dieting, control hunger, and gain muscle effectively.

• Eating enough carbs helps you perform better in your workouts and gain muscle faster.

• Eating enough fat promotes a healthy hormone profile, helps you better absorb the nutrients you eat and have healthy skin and hair.

• That's why you have to do more than getting your calories right. You have to get your "macros" right, too (eat the right amounts of protein, carbs, and fat).

And how do you do that, exactly?

Let's start by figuring out your protein intake.

• If your goal is to lose fat, research shows that you should eat about 1 to 1.2 grams of protein per pound of body weight per day for the best results.

If you're very overweight (25%+ body fat in men and 30%+ in women), then you can drop your protein intake to 1 gram per pound of lean body mass.

• If you want to gain or maintain your weight, then 1 gram of protein per pound of body weight per day is sufficient.

You should then calculate your fat intake next.

• If you want to lose fat, eat between 0.2 and 0.25 grams of fat per pound of body weight per day.

• For maintenance or muscle gain, bump that up to 0.3 to 0.35 grams per pound per day.

That leaves your carbs, which should simply comprise your remaining calories for the day (30 to 50% of total daily calories for most people).

Step 4. Create a meal plan that works.

Your efforts to build your best body ever can be thwarted by stupidly simple things.

Not having the right foods at home, for example. Or being too restrictive with the foods you "allow" yourself to eat. Or accidentally eating more calories that you mean to.

That's why I recommend you become skilled at meal planning. It's the simplest way to guarantee results in the gym.

A meal plan is exactly what it sounds like: a plan for what you're going to eat and when.

It doesn't have be boring, restrictive, or inconvenient, either. In fact, a good meal plan is the complete opposite. You should look forward to your meals, you should eat the foods you like, and it should never feel burdensome.

Step 5. Train while fasted.

At this point, you may be wondering how exercise fits into all of this.

Well, many people that do intermittent fasting also do a lot of "fasted training."

Many people mistakenly think these are the same thing, but they're not. When we're talking intermittent fasting, we're talking about when we eat. Fasted training, on the other hand, is when we exercise.

Basically, if you exercise after having fasted (real fasting, by the way–no food or calories) for 5 to 6 hours, it's fasted training.

Your insulin levels are low, and your body is relying solely on its power stores to stay alive.

On the other hand, if you exercise after having eaten in the last few hours, it's "fed" training because insulin levels are lofty and your body is running at least partly on energy obtained from the meal.

Now, you don't have to train while fasting if you're doing IF (you can work out after breaking your fast), but you may find it more convenient.

Many people doing IF like to work out first thing in the morning, and break their fasts afterward with a big post-workout meal.

Many people also like to do fasted training while cutting, because it helps you burn more fat in your workouts, and especially "stubborn fat" that clings to your abs, hips, and thighs.

You can also combine it with a few supplement to further amplify these fat-burning advantages.

CHAPTER 8: TIPS & TRICKS FOR WOMAN OVER 50 STARTING INTERMITTENT FASTING

Fasting For Weight Loss

There are new weight loss plans coming out every day from all around the world. With so many of these new diets and ideas, how can we be sure of which one's work and which ones do not? We simply cannot, and that is the case with the idea of fasting for weight loss. Hearing this now may sound silly, but we should definitely be questioning fasting as an effective means of weight loss because it seems reasonable.

We know that in order to lose weight, you have to be at some sort of calorie deficit. It is simple as that. You will lose weight if you consume less than your use. So with this principle, we would think that fasting would be a great means of dieting because you will be at a great calorie deficit while still having the same calorie use assuming you continue doing the same activities every day.

The truth is, fasting can be effective to some notch or another. It all depends how far you are really taking this process. If you are going to the point of starvation, then fasting will not work. It will simply put too much strain on your body, and it will begin to shut down. As it is shutting down, it goes into fat storing mode.

This means that most anything that you eat from that point forward, if not used immediately, will be converted into fat. This fat will then be stored where ever the body feels is the most fitting.

If by fasting you mean cutting your caloric intake abstemiously, then the fasting for weight loss diet will work for you. Assuming that you still have two to three small meals a day with adequate fluid intake, you would be losing weight in no time.

Because your body will burn around 2000 calories a day normally, this diet will have you burning twice as many calories as you consume. Over the course of a week, this will help you cuts as much as two pounds alone.

You can even add additionally to what you may already be burning through fasting for weight loss. You can take part in other diets such as the fruit juice diet. What is can do is cleanse your system and help clean out some of the excess water that your system is storing for no reason.

You can also add exercise to your calorie deficit to explode your weight loss. Just make sure to get the major food groups and vitamins and minerals every day!

"Fasting for weight loss", is probably the most ignored method of losing weight, yet it has been proven to be a very successful substitute.

When most persons think about the whole idea of "fasting weight loss", they tend to shy away because they view it as too torturous and inhumane; while others view fasting as a fanatical practice only done by highly spiritual gurus.

"Effects of fasting" - what happens in your body when you fast?

When you fast, you abstain from food by drinking purely water (water fast) or natural fruit juice (juice fast), in order to allow the body to initiate its natural healing/cleansing mechanism, which is detoxification. Detoxification is a process by which the body eliminates or deactivates toxins form the colon, liver, kidney, lungs, lymph glands and skin.

When food is no longer entering the body, the body turns to fat reserves for energy, these fat reserves were created when excess glucose and carbohydrates were not used for energy or growth, or excreted, so are therefore converted into fat. When these fat reserves are used for energy during a fast, it releases chemicals (toxins) which are then evicted through the above mentioned organs.

Though fasting detoxifies the body, it's also recommended that a "parasite cleanse" is done to have exact detoxification result.

Fasting - and not starvation

Another reason why people shy away from using fasting as a means to attain weight loss, they think it will make them starve to death or harm them in some other way.

The truth is, only improper fasting leads to starvation or cause other complications. Fasting is only harmful when done without liquid in-take or if persistent after hunger returns - when on a total fast. Hunger returning is an indication that all the fat reserves have been used up; usually occurs on a total fast which extends beyond three days. That intense hunger first felt will gradually leave after the first 24 - 36hrs, but returns when all the fat reserves have been completely used up, at this point the fast should be discontinued.

The first step before you begin your fasting

The first step I would urge you to do is to talk to your doctor, (but be warned, not all doctors are trained in this area and may possess limited understanding of fasting). But the wisest choice still, is to have a thorough check up (physical examination) to ensure you are in good health. By taking an examination, you may discover you have a physical condition that makes fasting unsafe or dangerous. And also, if you are on medication, be sure to have a talk with your doctor before making the step.

Examples of persons who should not fast without doctors' advice, and/or professional supervision

" Woman who are pregnant or nursing

" Anyone with tumors, bleeding ulcers, cancer, blood diseases, or heart disease

" If you suffer from chronic problem with kidneys, liver, lungs, heart, and other organs

" Persons who are taking insulin for diabetes, or suffer from other blood sugar problem such as hyperglycemia.

Even if you fall in the above mentioned category, don't be discouraged, like I said, first go and get a checkup from your doctor.

It would also be better if such persons' part-takes in a supervised "fasting weight loss" program, where the fasting is monitored by a trained individual (there are therapeutic fasting centers that offer this service for a charge). But remember to first check with your doctor before taking that route.

How does "fasting for weight loss" works?

When you fast, you take a break from the consumption of food thus giving your body a rest, allowing accumulated toxic waste matters to be removed. That's why liquid intake becomes necessary, because it speeds up the detoxification process allowing toxins to be eliminated and excreted from the body mainly through urination.

The byproduct of this method of detoxification is the removal and reduction of unhealthy body fat, hence producing significant weight loss.

How much weight can I expect to lose?

Weight loss through fasting depends on two things: how quick your body takes to purge itself, and the length of the fast. For some people, they will start seeing results in as little as three days, while with others, it may require a longer length of time or several phases of fasting to see significant weight reduction.

But to retain and maintain the obtained benefits of fasting weight loss, it is important that you first rid your body of parasite by taking a parasite cleanse, then stick to a balance and nutritious diet that will help you to have less toxic build up in your body allowing you to keep a stable weight.

Fasting for weight loss is without a doubt one of the best methods of losing weight, because it leads to the elimination of poisonous toxins from your body and restores your health; but as effective as it has proven to be, it should also be accompanied by a "parasite cleanse" to ensure the "benefits of fasting" isn't lost.

Fasting For Women

For women who are interested in weight loss, intermittent fasting may seem like a great choice, but many people want to know, should women fast? Is intermittent fasting effective for women? There have been a few key studies about intermittent fasting which can help to shed some light on this interesting new dietary trend.

Intermittent fasting is also known as alternate-day fasting, although there are certainly some variations on this diet. The American Journal of Clinical Nutrition performed a study recently that enrolled 16 obese men and women on a 10-week program.

On the fasting days, participants consumed food to 25% of their estimated energy needs. The rest of the time, they received dietary counseling, but were not given a specific guideline to follow during this time.

As expected, the participants lost weight due to this study, but what researchers really found interesting were some specific changes. The subjects were all still obese after just 10 weeks, but they had shown improvement in cholesterol, LDL-cholesterol, triglycerides, and systolic blood pressure.

What made this an interesting find was that most people have to lose more weight than these study participants before seeing the same changes. It was a fascinating find which has spurred a great number of people to try fasting.

Intermittent fasting for women has some beneficial effects. What makes it especially important for women who are trying to lose weight is that women have a much higher fat proportion in their bodies. When trying to lose weight, the body mainly burns through carbohydrate stores with the first 6 hours and then starts to burn fat. Women who are following a healthy diet and exercise plan may be struggling with tenacious fat, but fasting is a realistic resolution to this.

Intermittent Fasting for Women Over 50

Obviously our physiques and our metabolism changes when we hit menopause. One of the biggest transformations that women over 50 experience is that they have a slower metabolism and they begin to put on weight. Fasting may be a good way to reverse and prevent this weight gain though.

Research have shown that this fasting pattern assists to regulate appetite and people who follow it regularly do not experience the same cravings that others do. If you're over 50 and trying to adjust to your dimmer metabolism, intermittent fasting can help you to avoid eating too much on a day-to-day basis.

When you reach 50, your body also starts to develop some chronic diseases like high cholesterol and abnormal blood pressure. Intermittent fasting has been shown to decrease both cholesterol and blood pressure, even without a great deal of weight loss.

If you've started to notice your numbers rising at the doctor's office each year, you may be able to bring them back down with fasting, even without losing much weight.

Intermittent fasting may not be a great idea for every woman. Anyone with a specific health condition or who tends to be hypoglycemic should consult with a doctor. However, this new alimentary trend has specific benefits for women who naturally store more fat in their bodies and may have trouble getting rid of these fat stores.

Both men and women scuffle with weight problems. However, women are more eager when it comes to keeping their looks. It is the dream of every woman to have a perfect body that looks good in any and every clothing.

This makes losing weight more serious for women as they want to look their best at all times. The good news about losing weight is that there are several methods to make the process faster and easier.

Limit Calorie Intake

The one thing that needs to be understood clearly when it comes to losing and adding weight is that the calories are the main culprits. If you end up eating more calories than you burn, then you end up gaining weight. This makes it very important to make sure that the calories in are less than the calories out. You can simply accomplish this by restraining the amount of calories that you eat on a daily basis. It means knowing your foods and their calorie levels followed by getting the portions right. You then must make sure that you burn more calories daily. It is the secret on how to lose weight fast for women.

Move More

The accuracy is that most career women barely find time to move around. They are in most cases swamped in the office and take only very short breaks. However, easy walks can do the magic for you when it comes to losing weight. Even when at the office, try and walk about more. You can take benefit of your breaks to go for short walks which will fetch you great results with losing weight. When you are on the move, you boost the natural rate of metabolism which keeps the fats burning.

The more dynamic you are throughout the day the better it will be for your weight loss goals.

Workout Regularly

Working out seems like a lot of work. The truth however is that there are very simple exercises that you can do even without having to stay at the gym. When you keep up with a regular workout regime, you will be increasing the chances of losing weight fast. You can do a run or if you have time, spend a few minutes in the gym several times a week. Working out does not only ensure that fat is kept burning at a high level, but it also helps in toning your body.

Focus More on Intense Cardio

Cardio exercises have never disappointed when it comes to losing weight. You might therefore find it more beneficial to focus especially on intense cardio sessions. They provide a simple way of elevating the metabolism and burning calories. The best thing about cardio exercises is that the activities are fun and exciting. You will therefore enjoy your sessions more thus getting most out of it. Some of the intense exercises that you can focus on include indoor riding, running, swimming and gap training.

CHAPTER 9: HOW TO OVERCOME DOWN MOMENTS DURING INTERMITTENT FASTING

Tip 1: Gradually stretch out the number of hours you go between meals until you reach a 12-hour eating window. Then move to a 10-hour eating window and reduce by small increments until you reach your goal.

Tip 2: Plan ahead. Prepare a healthy meal that's ready for you when your fast ends and make sure to eat whole ingredients when possible including healthy carbs like whole grains, lean protein and plenty of veggies, says Fung.

Tip 3: Track your hydration using an app like MyFitnessPal, which can help keep you accountable and stick to water, plain tea or black coffee while fasting.

Tip 4: "Gradually change your diet along with your eating schedule by incorporating healthier foods slowly," suggests Stephens. This prevents you from trying to overhaul everything at once, which is more sustainable.

Tip 5: Keep up with your usual workout routine or try something low-impact like walking. If you fast overnight and exercise in the morning, you can eat a protein-rich meal after, which helps you increase the rate at which you build muscle.

Tip 6: Shift your schedule forward or backward by a few hours on days when you've got plans with friends so you can still enjoy socializing. "It's a lifestyle, and it has to fit into life's special occasions," An expert says. "Intermittent fasting can be flexible."

Intermittent fasting is pretty simple.

At bottom, you don't eat for most of the day, then you cram all of your calories into an "eating window" that can last anywhere from a couple to 6 to 8 hours.

If that sounds stupid, uncomfortable, or even unhealthy, I understand. I thought the same thing when I first heard about it years ago.

It turns out, though, that it's not like other fad diets. It's not going to go the way of the grapefruit diet, "detox" cleanses, and the dodo bird.

On the contrary, intermittent fasting can be an effective tool for refining nutritional compliance, it has good science on its side, and it doesn't have to be unpleasant.

In fact, many people enjoy IF more than traditional eating patterns, mainly because it allows you to have larger meals.

What IF isn't, though, is a phenomenon maker.

It won't automagically help you gain muscle and lose fat at the same time, burn away that belly fat, or stay young forever.

As you'll learn in this book, the fundamentals of appropriate dieting still very much apply, and the main reason to do it is simply because you like it.

CHAPTER 10: GUIDE OF FOODS TO EAT AND TO AVOID

The Basics of eating on Intermittent Fastin

There may be a lot of readers who are only familiar with one or the other. Both have a special style that packs a big punch to fat loss and proper health. On the surface only one of them is considered a "diet," but even that term is held very loosely. I am very familiar with both of them in regards to fat loss and overall health benefits so to give an overall summary for both will be suitable. I truly believe that if you bridge the gap and combine these two styles, you will be able to produce some pretty amazing fat loss results. Let's begin!

Fasting for Fat Loss Is Extremely Effective

The idea of fasting in a diet plan tends to get very negative remarks within the fitness culture. Many companies and trainers have us believing that if you aren't eating every few hours than your metabolism will slow down or cause our bodies to go into "starvation mode." Before we go any further, we must establish that "slowing of the metabolism" may be one of the biggest myths in the entire fitness industry. Metabolism is decreased under chronic, low-calorie consumptions that last weeks on end.

This does not happen when fasting is done a couple times a week. Here is a simple outline of how intermittent fasting is applied into someone's schedule. I'll explain how this can be tweaked to your liking later.

1. Eat normal until dinner (2-4 meals, not 6-8)

2. Eat your dinner but stop eating after that.

3. Fast until dinner the following day. (No calorie consumption)

4. For that meal just eat a regular size dinner.

In this approach you are still fasting for a 24-hour period, but are still having a meal every day. This is done typically 1-2 times a week. If you need to drop a lot of weight before a vacation or reunion, then you can fast 3 times a week. I would only recommend this for a few weeks.

What You Learn About Yourself During Fasting

When fasting, you will want to take note of any changes in the way you eat. Once you have completed a 24 hour fast a few times, the reasons of what, when, and why you eat may be revealed to you. A lot of the reasons why we eat is because of emotional connections or pure habit and not with actual hunger itself. Sometimes we are so conditioned to eat at certain times that we consume a meal when we aren't hungry.

Intermittent Fasting Is a Lifestyle And Not A Diet

The reason why it is not considered a "diet" is because it doesn't restrict you to certain foods, recipes, combinations, instructions, or charts to follow in order to lose weight. It rids you of neurotic compulsive eating habits and allows you variety. Instead of completely avoiding a particular food because someone told you to, adding a variety of foods will actually prevent you from over-eating any type of "bad" food. Now that we have established this area of fat loss, let's turn to a deeper issue in regards to diet and health.

What Is the Phase One Diet AKA The Fungus Link?

Doug Kaufmann is the mastermind behind the idea of fungus and yeast contributing to bad health and weight loss failures. He has researched and documented how fungi produces venomous substances called "mycotoxins" which causes many health problems. He tackles the problem by addressing areas where fungi and yeast can enter the body, but also provides the solution in starving the fungus to reverse the symptoms of so many health problems in America.

He has found that fungi, like people, crave specific carbohydrates. Knowing that fungi must have carbohydrates in order to thrive inside the body makes the Phase 1 Diet understandable to use.

So What Is Allowed On the Phase 1 Diet?

This is the only "diet" that I would ever recommend that actually restricts certain types of food, but for a specific reason. The exclusion of certain foods is done momentarily to starve and kill the fungus as well as exposing the root of food cravings. Food cravings that are not under control can be detrimental to your health as well as the added pounds on the belly, thighs, hips, you name it.

Fungus overgrowth may in fact be the root failure in losing the weight. As long as you are addicted to certain foods you will continue to eat and eat unconsciously. Many people find that their health elevates to a level where they can't believe how great they feel. A large reason for this is because of the specific food choice that starves and prevents overgrowth of fungus. Many people are living better because of this breakthrough approach to eating. Here is a quick outline of food choices that are suitable on the Phase 1 Diet.

Example of Acceptable Foods for The Phase 1 Diet

1) Eggs

2) Fruit: Berries, Grapefruit, Lemon, Lime, Green Apples, Avocado, Fresh Coconut

3) Meats: Virtually all meat including fish, poultry and beef

4) Vegetables: Fresh, unblemished vegetables and freshly made vegetable juice

5) Beverages: Bottled or filtered water, non-fruity herbal teas, stevia sweetened fresh lemonade, freshly squeezed carrot juice.

6) Vinegar: apple cider vinegar

7) Oils: olive, grape, flax seed, cold pressed virgin coconut oil

8) Nuts: raw nuts, including pecans, almonds, walnuts, cashews, and pumpkin seeds. Stored nuts tend to gather mold, so be careful!

9) Sweetner: Stevia, Xylitol

10) Dairy: Organic Butter, Organic Yogurt, (use the following very sparingly) cream cheese, unsweetened whipping cream, real sour cream.

Types of foods for intermittent fasting

Of all the fad diets of the moment, intermittent fasting has garnered much attention for its convincing evidence in scientific literature. Throughout history, fasting has been utilized as an expression of political dissent, desire for spiritual reward, as well as a therapeutic tool, but only recently has it gained widespread traction among fitness gurus for its touted weight loss and anti-aging effects.

But that brings the big question: is there an ultimate intermittent fasting guide so you know what to eat while you're on this diet?

First, let's take a step back and break down the basics: How does the diet work when it comes to these major intermittent fasting health benefits?

Scientists postulate that the anti-aging benefits are largely due to increased insulin sensitivity, and weight loss is related to an overall reduced calorie intake because of a shortened feeding window. Simply put, when you have less time during the day to eat, you eat less. Easy, right? But a key concept, as with any diet, is determining feasibility for your lifestyle.

One recent The Lancet Diabetes & Endocrinology study showed diet-induced weight loss typically leads to a 70 percent regain in weight, so finding any type of weight-loss plan that works best for you and won't cause you any destruction in the future is the key.

Fasting from 9 p.m. until about 1 p.m. the next day works well because most people are already skipping breakfast or are eating poor ones. This method can work well around a day job, but also emphasizes the importance of maintaining dietary needs around this time restricted feeding window.

This means that overall diet quality and habitual food choices still matter while intermittent fasting and that you probably won't get the body of your dreams while chowing down on nothing but hamburgers and fries.

In fact, eating junk food in a condensed feeding window on the IF diet may actually put you at risk of a shortfall of key nutrients such as calcium, iron, protein, and fiber, all of which are essential for normal biological function.

Plus, eating a diet rich in fruits and vegetables allows for more antioxidants in your body, which, like the metabolic effects of intermittent fasting, may subsidize to a longer lifespan!

For starters, here's a breakdown of typical intermittent fasting schedules:

• Alternate Day Fasting (ADF)—1-day ad libitum eating (normal eating) alternated with 1-day complete fasting

• Modified Alternate Day Fasting (mADF)—1-day ad libitum feeding alternated with 1 day very low-calorie diet (about 25 percent of normal caloric intake)

• 2/5—Complete fasting on 2 days of the week with 5 days' ad libitum eating

• 1/6—Complete fasting on 1 day of the week with 6 days' ad libitum eating

• Time Restricting Feeding (TRF)—Fasting for 12-20 hours per day (as a prolongation of the nighttime fast) on each day of the week. "Feeding window" of 4-12 hours.

OK, so you have the time windows for when you can chow down, but you're probably wondering what to eat during your IF journey. We rounded up 19 of the best foods to create the ultimate intermittent fasting food guide that will help prevent nutrient shortfalls!

1. Water

One of the most important aspects of maintaining a healthy eating pattern while intermittent fasting is to promote hydration. As we go without fuel for 12-16 hours, our body's preferred energy source is the sugar stored in the liver, also known as glycogen.

As this energy is burned, so disappears a large volume of fluid and electrolytes. Drinking 8+ cups of water per day will prevent dehydration and also promote better blood flow, cognition, and muscle and joint support during your intermittent fasting regimen.

2. Coffee

What about a warm cup of Joe? Will a daily Starbucks run break the fast? It's a common question among newbie intermittent fasters, but worry not: coffee is allowed.

Because in its natural state coffee is a calorie-free beverage, it can even technically be consumed outside a designated feeding window, but the minute syrups, creamers, or candied flavorings are added, it can no longer be consumed during the time of the fast, so that's something to keep in mind if you frequently doctor up your drink.

3. Minimally-Processed Grains

Carbohydrates are an essential part of life and are most definitely not the enemy when it comes to weight loss. Because a large chunk of your day will be spent fasting during this diet, it is important to think strategically about ways to get enough calories while not feeling overly full.

Though a healthy diet minimizes processed foods, there can be a time and place for items like whole grain breads, bagels, and crackers, as these foods are more quickly digested for fast and easy fuel. If you intend to exercise or train recurrently while intermittent fasting, these will especially be a great source of energy on the go.

4. Raspberries

Fiber the stuff that keeps you regular was named a shortfall nutrient by the 2015-2020 Dietary Guidelines, less than 10 percent of Western populations consume adequate levels of whole fruits. With 8 grams of fiber per cup, raspberries are a pleasant high fiber fruit to keep you regular during your shortened feeding window.

5. Lentils

This wholesome superstar packs a high fiber punch with 32 percent of total daily fiber needs met in only half a cup. Additionally, lentils provide a good source of iron (about 15 percent of your daily needs), another nutrient of anxiety, especially for active females undergoing intermittent fasting.

6. Potatoes

Similar to breads, white potatoes are digested with minimal effort from the body, and if paired with a protein source, they are a perfect post-workout snack to refuel hungry muscles. Another grant making potatoes an indispensable staple for the IF diet is that once cooled, potatoes form a resistant starch primed to fuel good bacteria in your gut.

7. Seitan

The EAT-Lancet Commission recently released a report calling for a dramatic reduction in animal-based proteins for optimal health and longevity. One large study directly linked consumption of red meat to increased mortality.

Make the most of your anti-aging fast by incorporating life-extending plant-based protein substitutes like seitan. Also known as "wheat meat," this food can be battered, baked, and dipped in your favorite sauces.

8. Hummus

One of the creamiest and tastiest dips known to mankind, hummus is another excellent plant-based protein and is a great way to boost nutritional content of staples like sandwiches (just sub for mayonnaise!) If you're courageous enough to make your own, don't forget the secret to the perfect recipe is ample garlic and tahini.

9. Wild-Caught Salmon

If your goal is to be a member of the centenarian club, you might want to read up on the Blue Zones. These five geographical regions in Europe, Latin America, Asia, and the U.S. are well known for dietary and lifestyle choices linked to extreme longevity. One commonly consumed food across these zones is salmon, which is high in brain-boosting omega-3 fatty acids EPA and DHA.

10. Soybeans

As if we needed another excuse to splurge for an appetizer at the sushi bar, is flavones, one of the active compounds in soybeans, have verified to inhibit UVB induced cell damage and stimulate anti-aging. So, next time you host a dinner party in, astonish your guests with a delicious recipe featuring soybeans!

11. Multivitamins

One of the proposed mechanisms behind why IF leads to weight loss is due to the fact that the individual simply has less time to eat and therefore eats less. While the principle of energy in versus energy out holds true, something that isn't often discussed is the risk of vitamin shortages while in a caloric deficit. Though a multivitamin is not necessary with a balanced diet of plenty of fruits and vegetables, life can get hectic, and a supplement can help fill the gaps.

12. Smoothies

If a daily supplement doesn't sound appealing, try springing for a double dose of vitamins by creating homemade smoothies packed with fruits and vegetables. Smoothies are a great way to consume multiple different foods, each uniquely packed with different essential nutrients.

Quick tip: Buying frozen can help save money and ensure ultimate freshness.

13. Vitamin D Fortified Milk

The recommended intake of calcium for an adult is 1,000 milligrams per day, or in plain speak, 3 cups of milk per day. With a reduced feeding window, chances to drink this much might be scarce, and so it is important to prioritize high calcium foods. Vitamin D fortified milk enhances the body's absorption of calcium and will help to keep bones strong.

To boost daily calcium intake, you can add milk to smoothies or cereal, or even just drink it with meals. If you're not a fan of the beverage, non-dairy sources high in calcium include tofu and soy products, as well as leafy greens like kale.

14. Red Wine

A glass of wine and a night of beauty sleep may keep heads turning, as the polyphenol found in grapes has distinct anti-aging effects. Humans are known to have one of the enzyme classes SIRT-1, which is thought to act upon resveratrol in the presence of a caloric deficit to enhance both insulin sensitivity and longevity.

15. Blueberries

Don't let their miniature size fool you: Blueberries are proof that good things come in small packages! Studies have shown that longevity and youthfulness is a result of anti-oxidative processes. Blueberries are a great source of antioxidants and wild blueberries are even one of the highest sources of antioxidants. Antioxidants help rid the body of free radicals and prevent widespread cellular damage.

16. Papaya

During the final hours of your fast, you'll likely start to feel the effects of hunger, especially as you first start intermittent fasting. This "hanger" may, in turn, cause you to overeat in large quantities, leaving you feeling bloated and lethargic minutes later. Papaya possesses a unique enzyme called papain that acts upon proteins to break them down. Including chunks of this tropical fruit in a protein-dense meal can help ease digestion, making any bloat more manageable.

17. Nuts

Make room on the cheese board for a mixed assortment, because nuts of all varieties are known to rid body fat and lengthen your life. A prospective trial published in the British Journal of Nutrition even associated nut consumption with a reduced risk of cardiovascular disease, type 2 diabetes, and overall mortality.

18. Ghee

Of course, you've heard a drizzle of olive oil has major health benefits, but there are plenty of other oil options out there you can use, too. You don't want to heat an oil you're cooking with beyond its smoke point, so next time you're in the kitchen whipping up a stir-fry, consider using ghee as your oil of choice. Basically just clarified butter, it has a much higher smoke point making it a great choice for hot dishes.

19. Homemade Salad Dressing

Just like your grandmother kept her cooking wholesome and simple, so should you when it comes to salad dressings and sauces. When we opt to make our own simple dressings, unwanted additives and extra sugar are avoided.

In fact, according to a dermatological journal, sugar might be accelerating the aging process more than any other ingredient by degrading cross-linkages of collagen fibers in our skin.

CHAPTER 11: TRAINING PROGRAM TO LOSE WEIGHT

Many people will ask if it is safe to combine fasting with exercise. I am here to say it is. However, some factors need to be considered before combining the two. First, the type of fasting regimen should be considered alongside the physical, mental, and psychological health of the individual. Women with existing medical conditions should not combine fasting with exercises before being advised by a medical expert. So, while it is safe to practice intermittent fasting and include exercise if you are an already active person, doing so is not suitable for everyone.   First of all, your metabolism can be negatively impacted if you exercise and fast for long periods. For example, if you exercise daily while fasting for more than a month, your metabolic rate can begin to slow down. So, while it may sound like a quick way to reap the benefits of your limited calorie intake, moderation is crucial. Combining the two can trigger a higher rate of breaking down glycogen and body fat. This means that you burn fat at an accelerated rate. Also, when you combine these two, your growth hormones are boosted. This results in improved bone density. Your muscles are also positively impacted when you exercise. Your muscles will become more resilient to stress and age slower. This is also a quick way to trigger autophagy keeping brain cells and tissues strong, making you feel and look younger.

Exercise is Even Better After 50

Cardiovascular exercise is great for the heart and lungs. It improves oxygen delivery to specific parts of your body, reduces stress, improves sleep, burns fat, and improves sex drive. Some of the more common cardio exercises are running, brisk walking, and swimming. In the gym, machines such as the elliptical, treadmill, and Stairmaster are used to help with cardio. Some people are satisfied and feel like they've done enough after 20 minutes on the treadmill, but if you want to continue to be strong and independent as you grow older, you need to consider adding strength training to your workout. After 50, strength training for a woman is no longer about six-pack abs, building biceps, or vanity muscles. Instead, it has switched to maintaining a body that is healthy, strong, and is less prone to injury and illness.   Women over 50 who engage in strength training for 20 to 30 minutes a day can reap the following benefits:

- Reduced body fat: Accumulating excess body fat is not healthy for any woman at any age. To prevent many of the diseases associated with aging, it is important to maintain healthy body weight by burning excess fat.

- Build bone density: With stronger bones, accidental falls are less likely to result in broken limbs or a visit to the emergency room.

- Build muscle mass: Although you are not likely to be the next champion bodybuilder, strength training will make you an overall stronger woman who will carry herself with ease, push your lawnmower, lift your groceries, and perform all other tasks that require you to exert some strength.

-Significant less risk of chronic diseases: In addition to keeping chronic diseases away, strength training can also reduce symptoms of some diseases you may have, such as back pain, obesity, arthritis, osteoporosis, and diabetes. Of course, the type of exercises you do if you have any chronic disease should be recommended by your doctor.   -

-Boosts mental health: A loss of self-confidence and depression are some psychological issues that come along with aging. Women who keep themselves fit with exercises tend to be generally more self-assured and are less

Strength Training Exercises for Women Over 50

These ten-strength training exercises you can do right in the comfort of your home. All you need is a mat, a chair, and some hand weights of about 3-8 pounds. As you get stronger, you can increase the weight. Take a minute to rest before switching between each routine. Ensure that you move slowly through the exercises, breathe properly, and focus on maintaining the right form. If you start to feel lightheaded or dizzy during your routines, especially if you are performing the exercise during your fasting window, stop immediately.

Squat to Chair

This exercise is great for improving your bone health. A lot of age-related bone fractures and falls in women involve the pelvis, so this exercise will target and strengthen your pelvic bone and the surrounding muscles.

To perform this:

1) Stand fully upright in front of a chair as if you are ready to sit and spread your feet shoulder-width apart.

2) Extend your arms in front of you and keep them that way all through the movement.

3) Bend your knees and slowly lower your hips as if you want to sit on the chair, but don't sit. When your butt touches the chair slightly, press into your heels to get back

your initial standing position. Repeat that about 10 to 15 times.

Forearm Plank

This exercise targets your core and shoulders.

Here's how to do it:

1) Get into a push-up position, but with your arms bent at the elbows such that your forearm is supporting your weight.

2) Keep your body off the mat or floor and keep your back straight at all times. Don't raise or drop your hips. This will engage your core. Hold the position for 30 seconds and then drop to your knees. Repeat ten times.

Modified Push-Ups

This routine targets your arms, shoulders, and core.

How's how to do it:

1) Kneel on your mat. Place your hands on the mat below your shoulders and let your knees be behind your hips so that your back is stretched at an angle.

2) Tuck your toes under and tighten your abdominal muscles. Gradually bend your elbows as you lower your chest toward the floor.

3) Push back on your arms to press your chest back to your earlier position. Repeat as many times as is comfortable.

Bird Dog

When done correctly, this exercise can strengthen the muscles of your posterior chain as it targets your back and core. It may seem easy at first, but can be a bit tricky.

To do this correctly:

1) Go on all fours on your mat.

2) Tighten your abdominal muscles and shift your weight to your right knee and left hand. Slowly extend your right hand in front of you and your left leg behind you. Ensure that both your hands and legs are extended as far as possible and stay in that position for about 5 seconds. Return to your starting position. This is one repetition. Switch to your left knee and right hand and repeat the movement. Alternate between both sides for 20 repetitions.

Shoulder Overhead Press

This targets your biceps, shoulders, and back.

To perform this move:

1) With dumbbells in both hands, stand and spread your feet shoulder-width apart.

2) Bring the dumbbells up to the sides of your head and tighten your abdominal muscles.   Slowly press the

dumbbells up until your arms are straight above your head. Slowly return to the first position. Repeat 10 times. You can also do this exercise while sitting.

Chest Fly

This targets your chest, back, core, and glutes.

To do this:

1) Lie with your back flat on your mat, your knees at an angle close to 90 degrees, and your feet firmly planted on the floor or mat.

2) Hold dumbbells in both hands over your chest. Keep your palms facing each other and gently open your hands away from your chest. Let your upper arms touch the floor without releasing the tension in them.

3) Contract your chest muscles and slowly return the dumbbells to the initial position. Repeat about ten times.

Standing Calf Raise

This exercise improves the mobility of your lower legs and feet and also improves your stability.

Here's how to perform it:

1) Hold a dumbbell in your left hand and place your right hand on something sturdy to give you balance.

2) When you are sure of your balance, lift your left foot off the floor with the dumbbell hanging at your side. Stand

erect and move your weight such that you are almost standing on your toes.

3) Slowly return to the starting position. Do this 15 times before switching to the other leg and doing the same thing all over again.

Single-Leg Hamstring Bridge

This move targets your glutes, quads, and hamstrings.

To do this:

1) Lie flat on your back. Place your feet flat on the floor or mat and spread your bent knees apart.

2) Place your arms flat by your side and lift one leg straight.

3) Contract your glutes as you lift your hips into a bridge position with your arms still in position. Hold for about 2 to 3 seconds and drop your hips to the mat. Repeat about ten times before switching your leg. Do the same again.

Bent-Over Row Bent-Over Row

This targets your back muscles and spine.

To do this:

1) Hold dumbbells in both hands and stand behind a sturdy object (for example, a chair). Bend forward and rest your head on the chosen object. Relax your neck and slightly bend your knees. With both palms facing each other pull

the dumbbells to touch your ribs. Hold the position for about 2 to 5 seconds and slowly return to the starting position. Repeat 10 to 15 times.

Basic Ab

A distended belly is a common occurrence in older women. This exercise can strengthen and tighten the abdominal muscles bringing them inward toward your spine.

To perform this:

1) Lie on your back with your feet firmly planted on the floor and your knees bent. Relax your upper body and rest your hands on your thighs.

2) As you exhale, lift yourself upward off the mat or floor. Stop the upward movement when your hands are resting on your knees. Hold the position for about 2 to 5 seconds and then slowly return to the starting position. Repeat for about 20 to 30 times.

Include Exercises in Your Daily Routine

You do not have to hit the gym or plan a time dedicated to working out. You can make exercise part of your daily routine so that you are always getting the proper amount of body movement, whether or not it is time for exercise. Here are a few tips on how to include exercises into your daily routine:

- Take the stairs (within reason) instead of using the elevator. You don't want to go up a ten-story building using the stairs! If you have a long way to go up or down, take the stairs a couple of flights and then complete your trip with the elevator.

- When you talk with your family members at home, don't shout from the top floor and bottom floor. Go up or climb down and talk with them.

- Find a sporting activity that you thoroughly enjoy and do it as often as is convenient. When you're doing something you enjoy, you'll hardly think of it as exercise, and you're likely to stay committed.

- If you are at work, instead of sending emails or text messages to coworkers, walk up to them and talk to them face to face.

- If possible, convert your one-on-one meetings to a walking meeting. Hold the meeting while taking a stroll outside.

- Stop a block or two from your destination and walk the rest of the way. Make walking your preferred mode of transportation.

- Take your dog for walks daily. If you don't have a dog, adopt one. It might seem that you are merely walking your dog, but you are exercising your muscles.

-Take brisk walks as often as possible. Remember to put on comfortable shoes when walking briskly. You can bring your walking shoes with you to make it easy for you to change into them.

CHAPTER 12: INTERMITTENT FASTING-FRIENDLY RECIPES

Egg Scramble With Sweet Potatoes

Servings: 1

Ingredients:

• 1 (8-oz) positive white colored potato, diced

• 1/2 cup reduce red onion

• 2 tablespoon cut rosemary oil

• Sodium

• Pepper

• 4 big eggs

• 4 significant egg whites

• 2 tablespoon sliced chive

Directions:

Preheat pot to 425 degrees F. Shake the interesting potato, salt, rosemary oil and reddish onion and pepper on a flat saucepan. Sprinkle with spray and roast until tender, approximately 20 minutes. Whip the potatoes, egg whites and a splash of salt and pepper together in a station cup. Sprinkle a fry pan with food spray preparation and scurry the agitate stations, about 5 minutes. Spray with chives cut and serve on spuds.

Every serving: 571 calories, 44 g of protein, 52 g of carbs (9 g thread), 20 g of excess fat.

Classical Chickpea Waffles Total Time: 30 minutes

Servings: 2

Ingredients:

• 3/4 cup chickpea flour

• 1/2 tbsp cooking soda

• 1/2 tablespoon sodium

• 3/4 cup ordinary 2% Greek yogurt

• 6 sizable eggs

To serve (optional), tomatoes, cucumbers, scallion, olive oil, parsley, yogurt and lemon extract, salt and onions.

Directions:

Oven preheat to 200 ° F. Place a cake rack over a piece of rimmed cooking, and put it in the cooktop. Warmth of a toaster oven in every way. Mix the flour, baking soda, and sodium into a sizable meal. In a tiny dish, combine yogurt and eggs together. Remove the damp ingredients straight into the ingredients completely dry out. Finishing toaster gently with spray of premium ready food items. In sets, reduce the combination of 1/4 to 1/2 cup in each component of the iron and gourmet chef to 4 to 5 minutes of golden brownish. The waffles transactions to the oven, and keep them comfortable. Standard with mix of stay. Serve waffles with a savory tomato mix, or a cozy almond butter and berries drizzle.

Every serving: 412 calories, 35 g of protein, 24 g of carbohydrates (4 g thread), 18 g of excess body fat.

Pb&J Overnight Oats

Servings: 1

Ingredients:

• 1/4 cup quick-cooking spun oats.

• 1/2 cup 2 per-cent dairy.

• 3 tablespoon velvety peanut butter.

• 1/4 cup mushed up raspberries.

• 3 tbsp entire raspberries.

Directions:

In a tool bowl, combine oatmeals, milk, peanut butter, and mushed up raspberries. Stir until smooth. Cover and amazing over night. In the morning, top and uncover with entire raspberries.

Every serving: 455 calories, 20 g protein, 36 g carbohydrates (9 g thread), 28 g excess fat.

Turmeric Extract Tofu Scramble

Servings: 1

Ingredients:

• 1 portobello mushroom.

• 3 or even 4 cherry tomatoes.

• 1 tbsp olive oil, plus a lot more for cleaning.

• Salt and pepper.

• 1/2 block (14-oz) agency tofu.

• 1/4 tsp ground turmeric remove.

• Dash garlic grain.

• 1/2 avocado, very finely sliced.

Directions:

Preheat oven to 400 ° F. Place the tomatoes and shroom on a baking sheet, and brush with oil. Sprinkle with salt and pepper. Roast for approximately 10 minutes, until tender. Meanwhile, mix the tofu, turmeric, garlic grain and a small volume of salt into a medium dish. Mash and a fork. Heat up 1 tbsp olive oil over low in a large saucepan. Add the tofu mixture and cook for about 3 minutes until firm and egg-like, stirring at regular intervals. Serve the tofu with mushroom, tomatoes and avocado and cover it.

Every serving: 431 calories, 21 g healthy protein, 17 g carbohydrates (8 g thread), 33 g fat.

Avocado Ricotta Power Toast

Servings: 1

Ingredients:

• 1 reduce whole-grain bread.

• 1/4 mature avocado, smashed.

• 2 tablespoon ricotta.

• Squeeze smashed reddish pepper scabs.

• Squeeze half-cracked ocean salt.

Directions:

Prepare your breadstuffs. Best of all with mango, ricotta, broken red pepper crusts and ocean salt. Eat with rushed, even hard-boiled eggs, plus a natural yogurt serving, or even fruit piece.

Per serving: 288 calories, 10 g healthy protein, 29 g carbs (10 g thread), 17 g body fat.

Turkish Egg Breakfast Total time

Servings: 2

Ingredients:

• 2 tbsp olive oil.

• 3/4 cup diced reddish alarm system pepper.

• 3/4 cup diced eggplant.

• Press each of salt and pepper.

• 5 huge eggs, carefully knocked.

• 1/4 tablespoon paprika.

• Diced cilantro, to taste.

• 2 blobs straightforward organic yogurt.

• 1 whole-wheat pita.

Directions:

Heat the olive oil in a medium-high, large, high-quality frying pan. Add pepper, sodium, eggplant, and pepper in the alarm. Sauce until relaxed, about 7 minutes. Interfere with taste with the eggs, paprika and extra salt and pepper. Prep, commonly mixing up until the eggs are slightly hurried. Sprinkle with decrease cilantro and serve with a ball of natural yogurt and the pita.

Every serving: 469 calories, 25 g healthy protein, 26 g carbohydrates (4 g thread), 29 g physical body excess fat.

Almond Apple Spice Muffins

Servings: 5

Ingredients:

• 1/2 stick butter.

• 2 cups almond food.

• 4 scoops vanilla protein particle.

• 4 sizable eggs.

• 1 cup unsweetened applesauce.

• 1 tablespoon sugar-cinnamon.

• 1 tbsp allspice.

• 1 tablespoon cloves.

• 2 tablespoon food preparation bit.

Directions:

Preheat the cooktop to 350 ° F. In a little bit of microwave-safe bowl, dissolve the butter in the microwave on small heat, concerning 30 secs. Mix all the remaining ingredients thoroughly with the dissolved butter. Spray 2 bun compartments with food preparation spray or dish linings for use with nonstick food. Put the mixture into the compartments of the muffin, ascertaining that it will not spill (3/4 full). This has 10 muffins to make. Place one shelf in the oven and make ready for 12 minutes.

Chicken Tacos

Servings: 4

Ingredients:

• 2 tsp oil.

• 1 little reddish onion, cut.

• 1 clove garlic, thoroughly cut.

• 1 pound. extra-lean ground chicken.

• 1 tablespoon sodium-free taco seasonings.

• 8 whole-grain corn tortillas, warmed up.

• 1/4 cup harsh lotion.

• 1/2 cup shredded Mexican cheese.

- 1 avocado, decrease.

- Condiment, for serving.

- 1 cup hairstyle lettuce.

Directions:

Heats up the oil in a big skillet on large outlets. Add the red onion and cook, blending for 5 to 6 mins until tender. Interfere with the garlic and beat for 1 min. Prepare the chicken and feed it, smash it with a spoon until almost brownish, 5 minutes. Add the seasonings with taco and 1 cup of tea. Simmer till deducted more than half, 7 mins. Fill out the tortillas with turkey and best with sour cream, cheese, condiment, lettuce, and avocado.

Every serving: 472 calories, 28 g of protein, 30 g of carbohydrates (6 g of fibre), 27 g of excess fat in the body.

Well-Balanced Spaghetti Bolognese

Servings: 4

Ingredients:

- 1 major pastas squash.

- 3 tbsp olive oil.

- 1/2 tablespoon garlic powder.

- Kosher salt and pepper.

- 1 tiny reddish onion, meticulously cut.

- 1 1/4 pound. ground chicken.

- 4 cloves garlic, finely cut.

- 8 oz. small cremini mushrooms, cut.

- 3 mugs fresh diced tomatoes (or also 2 15- oz canisters).

- 1 (8-oz) can quickly low-sodium, no-sugar- added tomato dressing.

- Fresh sliced up basil.

Directions:

Preheat the heating to 400 ° F. Sliced pastas squash lengthwise, and get rid of seeds. Massage every half with 1/2 tbsp of oil, and time with garlic particle and 1/4 tbsp of each salt and pepper. Blemish skin layer a top a rimmed food preparation item, and roast for 35 to 40 minutes until tender. Allow to cool down for 10 minutes. However, in a significant skillet on channel, cozy remaining 2 Tbsp oil. Add the onion, time with 1/4 tablespoon each salt and pepper, and prepare, mixing from time to time, till tender, 6 minutes. Add the chicken and prep, split it straight into a little sacrifice a spoon, 6 to 7 minutes till it is browned. Add the garlic and prepare 1 min. Move the mixture of chicken away from the pan, then add the mushrooms to the other. Chef, occasionally stirring, 5 mins until the mushrooms are tender. Interfere with the chicken. Add the dressing onions and tomatoes and simmer for 10 minutes. Take the squash as the sauce turns, and move to tables.

Spoon the Bolognese chicken over the very best and, if desired, dispersed with basil. Every serving: 450 calories, 32 g healthy protein, 31 g carbs (6 g string), 23 g physical body fat.

Chicken With Fried Cauliflower Rice

Servings: 4

Ingredients:

• 2 tablespoon grapeseed oil.

• 1 1/4 pound. boneless, skinless chicken boob, attacked to likewise thickness.

• 4 significant eggs, defeated.

• 2 reddish alarm peppers, carefully sliced.

• 2 small carrots, carefully diced.

• 1 onion, very carefully diced.

• 2 cloves garlic, properly diced.

• 4 scallions, finely cut, plus much more for serving.

• 1/2 cup frozen veggies, liquefied.

• 4 mugs cauliflower "rice".

• 2 tbsp low-sodium soy products sauce.

• 2 tablespoon rice white vinegar.

• Kosher sodium and pepper.

Directions:

Comfort 1 tablespoon of oil in a big, entrenched fry pan over medium-high. Add the chicken and plan for 3 to 4 moments each side until golden brownish. Transfer to a reduction board and allow for the remaining 6 minutes prior to slicing. Add 1 tbsp of remaining oil into the frying pot.Add the eggs and nationality for 1 to 2 moments, until just established; transfer to a recipe. Add the reddish onion, carrot, and pepper and cook alarm to the fry pan, mixing regularly until tender for 4 to 5 mins. Mix in the garlic and ready, 1 minutes. Shake with scallions and veggies. Add the cauliflower, soya products dressing, rice vinegar, salt and pepper and toss to mix. After that, allow the cauliflower rest, without blending, up until starting to brownish, 2 to 3 minutes. Shake with the sliced up chicken and eggs.

Every serving: 427 calories, 45 g healthy protein, 25 g carbs (7 g thread), 16 g excess body fat.

Piece Pan Steak

Servings: 4

Ingredients:

• A little bit of cremini mushrooms, trimmed and reduce in one- half.

• 1 1/4 lb. number broccolini, cut and reduce correct in to 2-in. lengths.

• 4 cloves garlic, properly cut.

• 3 tbsp olive oil.

• 1/4 tablespoon red pepper scabs (or also a bit additional for extra zest).

• Kosher salt and pepper.

• 2 1-in.- thick New York bit porks (about 1 1/2 lb total), reduce of excess fat.

• 1pc 15-oz may low-sodium cannellini surfaces, washed out.

Directions:

Preheat to 450 ° F the cooker. Toss the mushrooms, broccolini, garlic, oil, red pepper scabs and 1/4 tsp each salt and pepper on a large rimmed preparing food sheet. Place the piece of baking in the oven and roast for 15 mins. Push the skillet blend sideways to showcase the meats. Time the core in the skillet facility with 1/4 table spoon each salt and pepper and place. For medium-rare, toast the steaks to preferred doneness, 5 to 7 moments each tip. Moving the meat products to a reduced panel and allowing 5 minutes of rest before slicing. Add the grains to the food preparation slab and toss to include. Roast until heated via, around 3 mins. Serve surfaces and vegetables with steak.

Per serving: 464 calories, 42 g healthy protein, 26 g carbs (8 g thread), 22 g body system excess fat.

Pork Tenderloin With Squash Butternut And Brussels Sprouts

Servings: 4

Ingredients:

• 1 3/4 pound. pig tenderloin, trimmed.

• Sodium.

• Pepper.

• 3 tbsp canola oil.

• 2 sprigs fresh thyme.

• 2 garlic cloves, peeled off.

• 4 mugs Brussels sprouts, trimmed and cut in half.

• 4 mugs diced butternut squash.

Directions:

Heat up the device to 400 ° F. Season the tenderloin all over with salt and pepper. Heat energy 1 taste of oil higher over channel in a large cast iron skillet. Once the oil glows, sear and spread the tenderloin on all sides for 8 to 12 minutes until gold gray. On to a side. Add the thyme and garlic to the frying pan and stay 2 tbsp of oil, and chef for about 1 min, until odor is great. Fasten the sprouts in Brussels, squash with butternut and each sprinkle with a big salt and pepper. Prepare, mix regularly, for 4 to 6 moments, until the vegetables are a little brown. Find the tenderloin on top of the vegetables, and transmit to the oven every little thing. Roast until the injured vegetables and a meat product thermostat put right into the thickest part of the tenderloin shows 140 ° F, 15 to 20 minutes. Use cooktop gloves to remove the frying pan from the stove altogether. Before the veggies go up and serve, enable the tenderloin to rest about 5 minutes. Shake for edge feature with a vinaigrette dressing, eco-friendly.

Each serving: 401 calories, 44 g healthy protein, 25 g carbohydrates (6 g thread), 15 g body system excess fat.

Wild Cajun Spiced Salmon

Servings: 4

Ingredients:

• 1 1/2 lb. untamed Alaskan salmon fillet.

• Sodium-free taco seasoning.

• 1/2 scalp cauliflower (regarding 1 lb), separated flowers.

• 1 scalp broccoli (concerning 1 extra pound), separated florets.

- 3 tablespoon olive oil.

- 1/2 tablespoon garlic grain.

- 4 units. Tomatoes, diced.

Directions:

Preheat oven to 375 ° F. Put the salmon in a saucepan. In a little dish, combine the taco seasoning with 1/2 cup water. Area the mixture over the salmon, and bake till cloudy for 12 to 15 minutes. Pulse the cauliflower and cabbage in a food stuff cpu potato chip (in sets as needed), until properly cut and "riced". The oil warms up in a huge frying pan on the tool. Add the cauliflower and broccoli, scattered with garlic bit, and the chef, tossing for 5 to 6 moments until only tender. Serve salmon besides "rice" and finest with tomatoes.

For every serving: 408 calories, 42 g of protein, 9 g of carbohydrates (3 g of thread), 23 g of fat.

Pork Chops With Bloody Mary Tomato Salad

Servings: 4

Ingredients:

- 2 tablespoon olive oil.

- 2 tablespoon reddish white wine white colored vinegar.

- 2 tbsp Worcestershire sauce.

- 2 tablespoon ready horseradish, pressed completely dry.

- 1/2 tsp Tabasco.

- 1/2 tablespoon oats seeds.

- Kosher salt.

- 1 pint cherry tomatoes, halved.

- 2 oats stems, really very finely cut.

- 1/2 tiny reddish onion, very finely sliced.

- 4 tiny bone-in pig chops (1 in. slow-witted, involving 2 1/4 lb total amount).

- Pepper.

- 1/4 cup carefully diced flat-leaf parsley.

- 1 little scalp green-leaf lettuce, leaves behind torn

Directions:

Accurate to lead bigger barbecue. In a big tub, whip the butter, white vinegar, Worcestershire sauce, horseradish, Tabasco, celery seeds and 1/4 tbsp salt together. Shake the tomatoes, onion, and oatmeal with it. Season the pig chops with 1/2 tablespoon of each sodium and pepper, grill until perfectly browned, and prepare 5 to 7 minutes per edge just through. Fold the parsley right in to the tomatoes and serve over the veggies and pig. Eat with chopped cauliflower and even white potatoes.

For every serving: 400 calories, 39 g of protein, 8 g of carbs, 23 g of body fat.

Pb&J Overnight Oats

Servings: 1

Ingredients:

- 1/4 cup quick-cooking spun oats.

- 1/2 cup 2 per-cent dairy.

- 3 tablespoon velvety peanut butter.

- 1/4 cup mushed up raspberries.

- 3 tbsp entire raspberries.

Directions:

In a tool bowl, combine oatmeals, milk, peanut butter, and mushed up raspberries. Stir until smooth. Cover and amazing over night. in the morning, top and uncover with entire raspberries.

Every serving: 455 calories, 20 g protein, 36 g carbohydrates (9 g thread), 28 g excess fat.

Turmeric Extract Tofu Scramble

Servings: 1

Ingredients:

• 1 portobello mushroom.

• 3 or even 4 cherry tomatoes.

• 1 tbsp olive oil, plus a lot more for cleaning.

• salt and pepper.

• 1/2 block (14-oz) agency tofu.

• 1/4 tsp ground turmeric remove.

• dash garlic grain.

• 1/2 avocado, very finely sliced.

Directions:

Preheat oven to 400 ° f. Place the tomatoes and shroom on a baking sheet, and brush with oil. Sprinkle with salt and pepper. roast for approximately 10 minutes, until tender. Meanwhile, mix the tofu, turmeric, garlic grain and a small volume of salt into a medium dish. mash and a fork. Heat up 1 tbsp olive oil over low in a large saucepan. add the tofu mixture and cook for about 3 minutes until firm and egg-like, stirring at regular intervals. Serve the tofu with mushroom, tomatoes and avocado and cover it.

Every serving: 431 calories, 21 g healthy protein, 17 g carbohydrates (8 g thread), 33 g fat.

Avocado Ricotta Power Toast

Servings: 1

Ingredients:

• 1 reduce whole-grain bread.

• 1/4 mature avocado, smashed.

• 2 tablespoon ricotta.

• squeeze smashed reddish pepper scabs.

• squeeze half-cracked ocean salt.

Directions:

Prepare your breadstuffs. Best of all with mango, ricotta, broken red pepper crusts and ocean salt. Eat with rushed, even hard-boiled eggs, plus a natural yogurt serving, or even fruit piece.

Every serving: 288 calories, 10 g healthy protein, 29 g carbs (10 g thread), 17 g body fat.

Turkish Egg

Servings: 2

Ingredients:

• 2 tbsp olive oil.

• 3/4 cup diced reddish alarm system pepper.

• 3/4 cup diced eggplant.

• press each of salt and pepper.

• 5 huge eggs, carefully knocked.

• 1/4 tablespoon paprika.

• diced cilantro, to taste.

• 2 blobs straightforward organic yogurt.

• 1 whole-wheat pita.

Directions:

Heat the olive oil in a medium-high, large, high-quality frying pan. Add pepper, sodium, eggplant, and pepper in the alarm. Sauce until relaxed, about 7 minutes. Interfere with taste with the eggs, paprika and extra salt and pepper. Prep, commonly mixing up until the eggs are slightly hurried. Sprinkle with decrease cilantro and serve with a ball of natural yogurt and the pita.

Every serving: 469 calories, 25 g healthy protein, 26 g carbohydrates (4 g thread), 29 g physical body excess fat.

Almond Apple Spice Muffins

Servings: 5

Ingredients:

- 1/2 stick butter.

- 2 cups almond food.

- 4 scoops vanilla protein particle.

- 4 sizable eggs.

- 1 cup unsweetened applesauce.

- 1 tablespoon sugar-cinnamon.

- 1 tbsp allspice.

- 1 tablespoon cloves.

- 2 tablespoon food preparation bit.

Directions:

Preheat the cooktop to 350 ° f. In a little bit of microwave-safe bowl, dissolve the butter in the microwave on small heat, concerning 30 secs. Mix all the remaining ingredients thoroughly with the dissolved butter. Spray 2 bun compartments with food preparation spray or dish linings for use with nonstick food. Put the mixture into the compartments of the muffin, ascertaining that it will not spill (3/4 full). This has 10 muffins to make. Place one shelf in the oven and make ready for 12 minutes.

Chicken Tacos

Servings: 4

Ingredients:

• 2 tsp oil.

• 1 little reddish onion, cut.

• 1 clove garlic, thoroughly cut.

• 1 pound. extra-lean ground chicken.

• 1 tablespoon sodium-free taco seasonings.

• 8 whole-grain corn tortillas, warmed up.

• 1/4 cup harsh lotion.

• 1/2 cup shredded mexican cheese.

• 1 avocado, decrease.

• condiment, for serving.

• 1 cup hairstyle lettuce.

Directions:

Heats up the oil in a big skillet on large outlets. Add the red onion and cook, blending for 5 to 6 mins until tender. Interfere with the garlic and beat for 1 min. Prepare the chicken and feed it, smash it with a spoon until almost brownish, 5 minutes. Add the seasonings with taco and 1 cup of tea. Simmer till deducted more than half, 7 mins. fill out the tortillas with turkey and best with sour cream, cheese, condiment, lettuce, and avocado.

Every serving: 472 calories, 28 g of protein, 30 g of carbohydrates (6 g of fibre), 27 g of excess fat in the body.

Pork Tenderloin With Squash Butternut and Brussels Sprouts

Servings: 4

Ingredients:

• 1 3/4 pound. pig tenderloin, trimmed.

• sodium.

• pepper.

• 3 tbsp canola oil.

• 2 sprigs fresh thyme.

• 2 garlic cloves, peeled off.

• 4 mugs brussels sprouts, trimmed and cut in half.

• 4 mugs diced butternut squash.

Directions:

Heat up the device to 400 ° f. Season the tenderloin all over with salt and pepper. Heat energy 1 taste of oil higher over channel in a large cast iron skillet. Once the oil glows, sear and spread the tenderloin on all sides for 8 to 12 minutes until gold gray. On to a side. Add the thyme and garlic to the frying pan and stay 2 tbsp of oil, and chef for about 1 min, until odor is great. Fasten the sprouts in brussels, squash with butternut and each sprinkle with a big salt and pepper. prepare, mix regularly, for 4 to 6 moments, until the vegetables are a little brown. Find the tenderloin on top of the vegetables, and transmit to the oven every little thing. Roast until the injured vegetables and a meat product thermostat put right into the thickest part of the tenderloin shows 140 ° f, 15 to 20 minutes. Use cooktop gloves to remove the frying pan from the stove altogether. Before the veggies go up and serve, enable the tenderloin to rest about 5 minutes. Shake for edge feature with a vinaigrette dressing, eco-friendly.

Each serving: 401 calories, 44 g healthy protein, 25 g carbohydrates (6 g thread), 15 g body system excess fat.

Wild Cajun Spieced Salmon

Servings: 4

Ingredients:

• 1 1/2 lb. untamed alaskan salmon fillet.

• sodium-free taco seasoning.

• 1/2 scalp cauliflower (regarding 1 lb), separated flowers.

• 1 scalp broccoli (concerning   1 extra pound), separated florets.

• 3 tablespoon olive oil.

• 1/2 tablespoon garlic grain.

• 4 units. tomatoes, diced.

Directions:

Preheat oven to 375 ° f. Put the salmon in a saucepan. in a little dish, combine the taco seasoning with 1/2 cup water. Area the mixture over the salmon, and bake till cloudy for 12 to 15 minutes. Pulse the cauliflower and cabbage in a food stuff cpu potato chip (in sets as needed), until properly cut and "riced". The oil warms up in a huge frying pan on the tool. Add the cauliflower and broccoli, scattered with garlic bit, and the chef, tossing for 5 to 6 moments until only tender. Serve salmon besides "rice" and finest with tomatoes.

Every serving: 408 calories, 42 g of protein, 9 g of carbohydrates (3 g of thread), 23 g of fat.

CONCLUSION

With intermittent fasting becoming more and more popular as a weight-loss and health management diet, it is important to understand how to set it up; here are three keys to make sure that you can get involved in an intermittent fasting lifestyle as soon as possible.

Intermittent fasting doesn't need to be a short term approach to dieting and is in fact much more successful as a genuine lifestyle choice. The first decision to make therefore is how to adapt a fast to YOUR life. Remember that the fast can be anywhere from 16 hours to several days in length depending on exactly what you are trying to accomplish. The two approaches that are perhaps easiest to set up are an alternating day (24 hour) fast/eat cycle, or a 16/8 cycle.

When do I work out? This question is key. Diet is with doubt the most important factor in weight-loss and good health, but to really get the best out of an intermittent fast, the re-feed should coincide with your workout. Personally, I have had good success with a fast from 8Pm until the next day at lunch and an early afternoon training session. All the food that I am taking in around my workout is being used for fuel and to repair muscle rather than being stocked as body-fat.

What do I want to accomplish with intermittent fasting? Is your aim fat-loss, muscle gain, enhanced health or a combination of all three? Depending on your answer to these questions, you can start to identify exactly how long your fast should be and what quantity of food you should be eating during the eating "window".